HEMATOLOGY
LABORATORY
MANUAL

HEMATOLOGY LABORATORY MANUAL

By

Maurine J. Corsaut, M.S., M.T.(ASCP)SH, CLS

Assistant Professor, Department of
Health Sciences
Coordinator, Medical Technology Program
Illinois State University
Normal, Illinois

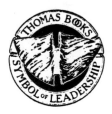

CHARLES C THOMAS • PUBLISHER
Springfield • Illinois • U.S.A.

Published and Distributed Throughout the World by

CHARLES C THOMAS • PUBLISHER

2600 South First Street

Springfield, Illinois 62717, U.S.A.

©*1982, by* CHARLES C THOMAS • PUBLISHER

ISBN 0-398-04524-0

Library of Congress Catalog Card Number: 81-5277

*With THOMAS BOOKS careful attention is given to all details of
manufacturing and design. It is the Publisher's desire to present books that are
satisfactory as to their physical qualities and artistic possibilities and
appropriate for their particular use. THOMAS BOOKS will be true to those
laws of quality that assure a good name and good will.*

Library of Congress Cataloging in Publication Data

Corsaut, Maurine J.
    Hematology.

    Bibliography: p.
    Includes index.
    1. Blood—Examination. 2. Hematology—Technique. I. Title. [DNLM:
1. Hematology—Laboratory manuals. WH 25 C826h]
RB45.C67   616.07'561   81-5277
ISBN 0-398-04524-0   AACR2

Printed in the United States of America
PS-RX-10

This book is dedicated to my students, past, present, and future. Each semester my life is renewed as a different group enters my classroom. My faith in mankind is revitalized by their enthusiasm and eagerness to learn. They are a stimulus that rekindles my enthusiasm and search for knowledge.

PREFACE

This book is written essentially for the student in clinical laboratory sciences. The material herein was written for the purpose of providing a laboratory reference for student medical technologists in a preclinical course in hematology. No other currently available manual provided the subject matter precisely desired by the author.

This book is not a manual of the whole field of hematological procedures, techniques, and theories. The theoretical material is provided to the extent necessary for understanding the concepts of the procedures and their results. It is hoped that persons using this manual will be able to perform the tests described and understand the material presented.

The procedures included in this book are essentially hand or semi-automated procedures. Although automated instruments are now used to perform most of the clinical laboratory analyses, training the laboratorian in manual procedures is still an essential component of the educational program and will remain so in the future. Development and mastery of manipulative skills and techniques are ultimately important in obtaining accurate and reliable results. These skills, once mastered, are easily adapted to those necessary for the operation of the most sophisticated instrumentation.

I wish to thank the artists at Charles C Thomas, Publisher for the illustrations appearing in this book; Mrs. Lenora Leicht for providing excellent typing skills during the preparation of this book; and Joan Polancic for her assistance with the original manuscript.

CONTENTS

Chapter *Page*

HEMATOLOGY
LABORATORY
MANUAL

---------- *Chapter 1* ----------

GENERAL LABORATORY PROCEDURES

OBJECTIVES

The student will learn the following:

1. the procedure for cleaning laboratory glassware.
2. the types of glassware used in the laboratory.
3. the procedures for the proper use of laboratory glassware (pipets specifically).
4. the parts of a microscope and how each is designed and used to achieve skill in microscopy.
5. the composition of blood.
6. the procedure for collecting blood by:
   a. microsampling
   b. venipuncture.
7. the types of anticoagulants and how they prevent coagulation of blood.

GLASSWARE

There are different types of glassware used in the clinical laboratory. Some types of glassware are designed to be used for specific purposes while other types may be used in routine procedures without specific designation. However, it is important that you understand the proper handling of each type.

Generally, there are two types of glassware used: the borosilicate type I glassware and the soda lime glassware. The borosilicate type is the less porous, very hard type of flint glass, which may be cleansed and reused. The soda lime glass is the porous, nonreusable type of glass that is designed to be used only one time and then discarded.

Cleaning Laboratory Glassware

If the borosilicate glassware is used, there are certain techniques in cleaning it that must be observed. The proper cleaning of this type of glassware is outlined below.

1. A *small* amount of detergent is placed in the washing receptacle and an adequate amount of water is added (too much detergent is difficult to rinse away).
2. The glassware is *thoroughly* washed.
3. The glassware is then thoroughly rinsed with tap water.

3

4. The glassware is next rinsed 3 times in distilled water.
5. It is then inverted to dry on the drying rack or placed in the drying oven.
6. It is replaced in its proper storage area.

Proper cleaning is *ultimately important* in maintaining the glassware free from contaminating materials from previous use or from the carry-over of detergent, which would cause inaccurate results during subsequent use.

Proper storage is also important to maintain glassware free from contaminants. Glassware should be stored in dust and chalk-free cabinets and drawers. Care must be taken that pipet tips do not become broken or chipped as this will result in inaccuracies in the pipet volume and flow-rate.

Using Laboratory Glassware

Glassware that is calibrated is designed to be used in a specific way. Improper use will affect the accuracy of the piece of glassware and, ultimately, the accuracy of the test being performed.

There are two types of pipets used in the laboratory: serological and volumetric.

Serological pipets are used in procedures that do not call for precise accuracy. There are reusable and disposable serological pipets. The disposable pipets are used only once and discarded because they are made of soda lime glass or other porous materials that absorb substances easily. Once used, these absorbed substances are difficult to wash away and may cause interfering reactions in other laboratory tests. Serological pipets are usually calibrated to within ±1 percent to ±5 percent accuracies.

Volumetric pipets are used when precise accuracy is indicated. Procedures that call for volumes of 1.0 ml, 0.1 ml, or 0.001 ml indicate accuracy is needed. Volumes of 1 ml, .5 ml, or 5 ml are not considered to be precise volumes and a serological pipet may be used to deliver these volumes. Volumetric pipets are more accurate than serological pipets because of the bulb. Less liquid retention to the surface of the internal bore of the pipet increases the accuracy of delivering a specified volume of liquid. There is less surface for retention of liquid in a volumetric pipet bulb.

Pipets are calibrated in the upright position. They are designed to be used in that manner if the accuracy is to be maintained. Holding the pipet at an angle will alter the flow rate, causing more retention of liquid to the inside of the pipet, thus altering the volume dispensed.

Pipets are designed to be used as To Deliver or To Contain.

To Deliver (T.D.) pipets are designed to deliver the volume indicated on the pipet. These pipets are either blow-out or drain-out pipets, depending upon the presence or absence of a frosted or painted ring or two rings at the top of the pipet. *Blow-out pipets* have a ring or rings at the top. They are calibrated to be used in the following way:

1. The solution is drawn to the calibration mark, or adjusted to the calibration mark.
2. Excess solution is wiped from the outside of the pipet in a downward motion, taking care not to pull any solution from inside the pipet.
3. The solution is allowed to drain out into the proper receptacle, keeping the pipet in the upright position.
4. The last drop of solution is then blown out.

Drain out pipets do not have a ring or rings at the top. They are calibrated to be used in the following ways:

1. The solution is drawn to the calibration mark, or adjusted to the calibration mark.
2. Excess solution is wiped from the outside of the pipet in a downward motion, taking care not to pull solution from inside the pipet.
3. The solution is allowed to drain out into the proper receptacle, keeping the pipet in the upright position.
4. The pipet is then touched to the edge of the receptacle, dispensing the remaining volume to be pipetted. (A small amount of solution will remain in the tip of the drain-out pipet. This is expected and is not a part of the volume to be delivered by the pipet.)

To Contain pipets are calibrated to be used *only when pipetting one solution into another solution.* They are always blow-out pipets. The procedure for using a To Contain pipet follows:

1. Solution I is drawn to the calibration mark, or adjusted to the calibration mark.
2. Excess solution is wiped from the outside of the pipet in a downward motion, taking care not to pull solution out of the pipet.
3. Solution I is allowed to drain out, or may be blown out, into solution II into which it is being pipetted.
4. Solution II is now drawn into the pipet 3 or 4 times to completely rinse solution I out of the pipet.
5. The last drop of solution I and II mixture is then blown out.

This procedure insures that the entire volume of solution I contained within the pipet has been dispensed into the second solution.

Careful attention to and use of the specific type of pipet called for in a laboratory procedure will increase the accuracy of the test being performed. Laboratories should always strive for accuracy in techniques. Proper use of laboratory glassware is no exception.

CARE AND USE OF THE MICROSCOPE

Microscopy is the skillful use of the microscope in a thorough and systematic manner for the investigation of a matter too small to be seen by the unaided eye.

Successful microscopy requires:

1. the use of a microscope mechanically and optically suited to the work at hand;
2. a knowledge of the basic principles of the microscope and its optical system;
3. skill in the use and care of the microscope;
4. an understanding of the nature of the material to be investigated, the method of preparation for examination, and the illumination required for adequate observation.

Obviously, then, there are many variables that must be controlled for successful microscopy. In order to accomplish this it is essential that you understand the relationship between (1) magnification, (2) resolving power, and (3) illumination.

Magnification

Magnification is the apparent increase in the size of an object.

Placing a convex lens between the eye and any object will result in magnification of that object, but certain other changes also take place in the relationship between the eye, the lens, and the object.

Light passing through the lens is refracted, determining the angle at which it enters the eye. The greater the curvature of the lens surface, the greater the angle of refraction, and the larger the object appears to be. Therefore, the greater the curvature of the lens, the higher the lens power.

Magnifying power of a single lens can be roughly calculated by using the following formula:

$10/f = $ *(magnifying power)*
where f = focal length in inches (the approximate distance between the lens and the object when the object is in sharp focus)

From the formula, we can see that the greater the focal length, the lower the magnifying power. Conversely, the higher the magnifying power the shorter the focal length.

The area of the object that can be examined through the lens is called the **field of view. As the focal length is reduced, the magnification is increased and the field of view is also reduced. Therefore, switching from a low power objective on the microscope to a higher power objective brings the objective closer to the object and also diminishes the field of view.**

Resolving Power

The resolving power of a microscope is the ability of the objective to distinguish fine detail in the specimen structure. It is indicated by the Numerical Aperture, or N.A., of the objective. It is defined as:

N.A. = n sin a
where n = the refractive index of the transparent medium (air, water, oil) between the objective lens and the object
a = the angle between the extreme marginal ray and the central ray entering the objective

N.A. is actually a mathematical rating based on the cone of light that an objective can utilize. The higher the N.A. of the objective, the greater the resolving power and the finer the detail it can reveal. The largest value for the size of an angle is 1; the refractive index of air is 1; the limit of N.A., when air is between the object and the objective lens is 1. If oil (or other fluid with an index of more than 1) is introduced between the objective and the object, we can obtain a greater value of N.A. and, consequently, can obtain higher resolving power and greater detail. The oil immersion objective can give greater resolution as well as higher magnification. To provide an illuminating cone with N.A. equal to that of the objective, oil must be substituted for air between the condenser and the slide. *We will only place the oil between the object and the objective lens, however.* (Figure 1)

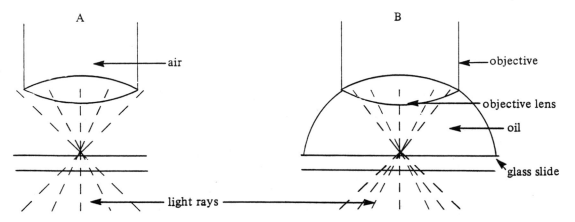

Figure 1. Light path through the high dry objective lens (A) and oil immersion objective lens (B). Redrawn from Barbara A. Brown: *Hematology, Principles and Procedures*, 2nd ed., 1976. Courtesy of Lea & Febiger, Philadelphia, Pennsylvania.

Illumination

The purpose of illumination is to light the specimen so that it can be seen to maximum advantage for significant examination. The more advanced the microscopy, the more important the source of illumination.

Objects are made visible to us because of the way they affect the light that reaches them from the sun, or from another source such as an incandescent lamp. An opaque object, for example, is recognized in form, color, or texture because of the light reflected from it to our eye. On the other hand, we recognize some objects by the way they affect the light that passes *through* them. They are more or less transparent, or appear as outlines against a luminous background.

Surface illumination for opaque matter (to make details visible by the light reflected into the microscope) and trans-illumination (making the structure visible by passing light through the matter) are the two forms of illumination for the microscope. The latter form is known as *bright field illumination* and is the principal method used for the examination of biological materials. (Other types of illumination include phase contrast, darkfield, and polarized light, but these will not be discussed.)

Proper utilization of the specific parts of your microscope designed to regulate the amount of light or create contrast is, therefore, ultimately important in order to attain successful microscopy.

Know Your Microscope

The first requirement in learning to use your microscope with maximum effectiveness is to know all of its parts, their correct names, and the proper functioning of each part.

Study the diagram (Figure 2) until you know all of the labeled parts.

Eyepiece Lens

The eyepiece lens has a magnification of 10X (X is used to designate the

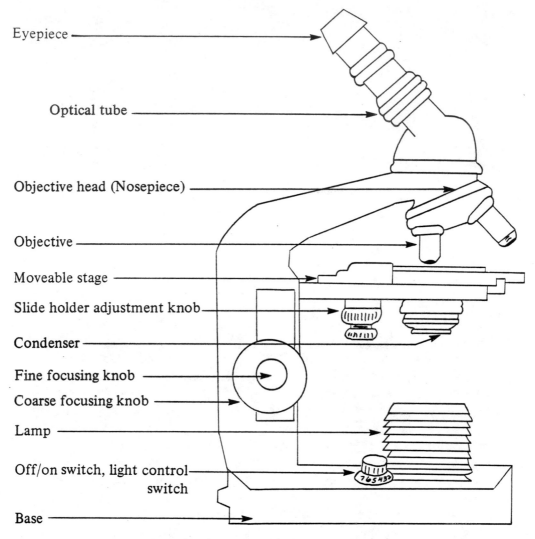

Eyepiece

Optical tube

Objective head (Nosepiece)

Objective

Moveable stage

Slide holder adjustment knob

Condenser

Fine focusing knob

Coarse focusing knob

Lamp

Off/on switch, light control
switch

Base

Figure 2. Microscope (Nikon® Binocular).

units of magnification known as diameters). This means that the lens magnifies the diameter of the object ten times its original size.

A monocular microscope has one eyepiece; a binocular microscope contains two eyepieces and is most commonly used today.

Objective Lens

Most clinical microscopes contain four objective lenses, each with different powers of magnification. The most commonly employed objectives are 10X (low power), 40X or 45X (high-dry), and 100X (oil immersion). An additional fourth lens, 4X may be used for scanning the specimen. The 10X objective is utilized to locate the specimen on the slide and is used for counting leukocytes in manual procedures. The 40X lens is used for counting erythrocytes and platelets by manual techniques. The 100X oil immersion is used for performing a differential count and blood smear examination. *It is extremely important that the immersion oil be used only in conjunction with the 100× lens* because this lens is the only one that has a protecting seal, which prevents the oil from entering the objective.

The total magnification is equal to the product of the magnification of the eyepiece lens and the magnification of the objective lens, i.e. 10× times 10× = 100×.

Optical Tube

The optical tube is the structure between the eyepiece and the objective lens. The aerial image is formed in this structure. The image formed is inverted, the object seen is upside down and reversed so that the right side of the object is seen at the left. Movement of the object is reversed also.

Nosepiece

The nosepiece holds the four objectives and rotates to facilitate changing from one objective to another. It permits parfocal adjustment during microscopy.

Moveable Stage and Slide Holder

The stage holds the slide within the slide holder and contains a moveable assembly, in order to facilitate the study of different parts of the slide. Movement is controlled by two small knobs located beneath the stage. Movement can be forward or backward, right or left.

Substage Condenser

The most commonly used substage condenser is the Abbe condenser, which functions to direct light from the source onto the specimen. It consists of two lenses. The light is focused on the object by raising or lowering the condenser system. Proper focusing is important to provide adequate and proper illumination for microscopy.

Iris Diaphragm

The iris diaphragm contains a number of leaves that may be opened or closed to increase or decrease the amount of light illuminating the specimen. It is located at the base of the substage condenser.

Light Source

A built-in light source is located in the base of the microscope. This is often housed within a structure called the lamp house. The light is directed up through the condenser system. There are controls for this illuminating system, enabling the user to increase or decrease the intensity of the light emanating from the bulb. This control is located on the base of the microscope.

Focusing Procedure

Right from the start is the way to focus properly. The procedure becomes automatic in a very short time, so doing it properly from the beginning means taking an easy step toward good microscopic technique.

1. Watching from the side of the stage, use the coarse adjustment to bring the stage up until the low power objective is about one-quarter inch above the slide.
2. Using the coarse adjustment, and looking through the eyepiece, lower the stage until the specimen comes into approximate focus. Proper illumination adjustment may be necessary also.
3. Using the low power objective, search the slide for various areas that are to be studied.
4. If higher magnification is needed for the procedure, turn the 40× objective into place (or 100× if need be).
5. Slight adjustment of the fine focus brings the object into sharp focus.

Eye Care

To enable comfortable use of the microscope for longer periods of time, the manufacturer has provided for adjustment of the interpupillary distance between the eyepieces. Grasp the two eyepieces and gently push them together or pull them apart until they are comfortable for you. There is also an adjustment within the left eyepiece to accommodate differences between the vision of the eyes. You may perform microscopy without eyeglasses unless you have astigmatism.

Care of the Microscope

Dust and dirt not only interfere with microscope efficiency but can actually be magnified to the point where they obscure or distort your view of the specimen. Make microscope cleanliness a habit from the start. Make it a point to inspect and clean your microscope before and after you use it until it becomes second nature. Some hints in cleaning:

1. Only lens paper should be used to clean the lenses. The paper is designed for this purpose and will not scratch the lenses as more harsh paper might.
2. Oil must be removed from the oil immersion lens (with lens paper) whenever it is not in use. Oil will harden, collect dust and dirt, and therefore, inhibit good microscopy.
3. The slide-holder should be turned so that the extension arm is not exposed during storage. Bumping the extension arm could cause the holder to be out of adjustment and interfere with proper slide manipulation.
4. Keep the microscope covered with the plastic cover when not in use.
5. Carry the microscope with two hands, and when placing it on a desk or table, do so with care. Avoid jarring it. Treat it like the precision instrument it is.

COMPOSITION OF BLOOD

Blood is a specialized form of connective tissue.

The total blood volume in an adult is approximately six liters ($6.0\pm1.0\ l$), or 7-8% of the body weight. Approximately 45 percent of this amount is composed of the formed elements of the blood: red blood cells, white blood cells, and platelets. The remaining 55 percent of the blood is the fluid portion, called *plasma*. Approximately 90 percent of the plasma is water; the remaining 10 percent is composed of proteins, carbohydrates, vitamins, hormones, enzymes, lipids, and salts.

If coagulation is prevented, the formed elements can be separated from the plasma. If blood is allowed to clot, the liquid portion exudes from the clot and this fluid is termed *serum*. The major difference between plasma and serum is that serum lacks fibrinogen and a few other coagulation factors, which are utilized to form the fibrin strands of the blood clot.

COLLECTION OF THE BLOOD SAMPLE

In order that blood may be studied or tested in various procedures, it must first be collected either by (1) microsampling (capillary puncture) or (2) venipuncture. The basis of hematological testing depends on the proper collection and handling of the blood sample in order to obtain reliable results.

Microsampling

Microsampling refers to blood collection from the finger, toe, heel, or earlobe, and will usually be done on patients in the following categories:
1. Newborn infants. The blood is generally obtained from the heel or big toe since these areas are larger than the fingertip.
2. Very young children. If only a small amount of blood is needed, the tip of the third or fourth finger is punctured.
3. Adults. In circumstances where the patient has very poor veins, or where the veins are not able to be used because of I.V. apparatus, the tip of the third or fourth finger may be used to obtain the blood.

Equipment and Reagents

1. alcohol, 70% or prepared alcohol (70%) swabs
2. dry sterile gauze pads or cotton balls
3. sterile blood lancet
4. appropriate pipets, diluting fluids, and micro-collecting tubes for tests ordered

Procedures

1. Using the appropriate finger, toe, etc., vigorously cleanse the puncture site with alcohol swab. (Vigorous cleansing will also increase circulation.)
2. Wipe area dry with sterile gauze or cotton.
3. Using the sterile lancet, make a deep puncture in the ball of the finger. (A deep puncture is no more painful than a superficial one, will give a better blood flow, and will make it unnecessary to repeat the puncture.)
4. Using the sterile gauze, wipe away the first drop of blood, making certain the area is completely dry. (The first drop that appears contains lymph and interstitial fluid, which dilute the blood.)

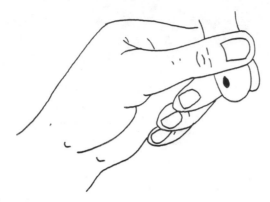

Figure 3. Site of fingertip puncture. Redrawn from Barbara A. Brown: *Hematology, Principles and Procedures*, 2nd ed., 1976. Courtesy of Lea & Febiger, Philadelphia, Pennsylvania.

5. Apply moderate pressure to obtain a drop of blood. Do not squeeze too tightly or tissue fluids will mix with the blood.
6. Release pressure immediately to allow recirculation of the blood.
7. **Collect the blood sample, repeating steps 5 and 6, if necessary, until blood is collected.**
8. **Apply a piece of gauze or cotton ball to the puncture site and use pressure until the bleeding has stopped.**

The values for the red blood count, hematocrit, hemoglobin, and platelets are somewhat lower in capillary blood than in venous blood. Whenever it is possible and the patient is old enough, a venipuncture should be performed.

Venipuncture

Larger volumes of blood needed for various clinical analyses are obtained from the veins of the forearm, wrist, or ankle. Because of conveniences and the larger size of the veins in the forearm, this area is usually chosen for a venipuncture.

A venipuncture must be performed with much care. Because there are a limited number of easily accessible veins in a patient, great care must be taken to preserve their good condition and availability.

The recommended procedure is to have the patient lying down. If this is not possible, he/she should be sitting in a sturdy, comfortable chair with his/her arm firmly supported on a table or chair arm and easily accessible to the technologist. The technologist must be prepared for the occasional patient who will faint during or following the venipuncture. Make certain that you do not place the collection tray where it could be upset by either the patient or yourself during the venipuncture procedure.

Equipment and Reagents

1. blood collection tray (phlebotomy tray)
2. requisition slip with patient's name, I.D. number, room, date, etc.

3. alcohol swabs (70% alcohol)
4. sterile gauze pads
5. Vacutainer® system (tubes, holder, needles) or sterile needles and appropriate syringes
6. plain and anticoagulated stoppered test tubes (if syringes are to be used)
7. test tube rack to hold tubes
8. wax pencil or pen to label collected blood samples
9. tourniquet

Vacuum Systems

Vacuum tubes are widely used today for blood collection. Rubber stoppers are color-coded to identify the anticoagulant present, or the tube may be kept plain and used for blood that will be allowed to clot. The vacuum within the tube is sufficient to draw a predetermined volume of blood. The system consists of a disposable double-pointed needle that screws into the holder. When the needle is in place, the vacuum tube is inserted in the holder and pushed onto the needle until the rubber stopper reaches the guide line. Care should be taken not to push the stopper beyond this line, or the vacuum will be released. Once the system has been assembled, the needle is inserted into the arm in the routine manner and the needle in the vacuum stopper is pushed through the diaphragm, breaking the vacuum and thus allowing the blood to flow into the tube. A prescribed amount of blood will flow into the tube and then the flow will stop. When more than one tube of blood is needed, the first tube may be removed from the needle and another inserted while the needle is still in the vein. Multiple samples may be drawn in this manner with only one venipuncture being done.

Needle and Syringe

The diameter or bore of the needle is indicated by its gauge number. The smaller the number, the greater the diameter. Gauges 20 and 21 are usually used for routine venipuncture.

The choice in size of syringe is regulated by the amount of blood needed for analysis. Ordinarily, a 10 ml syringe is most frequently used. Do not use a syringe in which there is any dampness. Moisture will hemolyze the blood. Plastic syringes are commonly used today. These are packaged in sterile packets and are disposable. If a glass syringe is to be used, its barrel and plunger must be matched.

When the needle and syringe have been removed from their packages, place the needle firmly onto the syringe. Do not handle the cannula of the needle. Keep the assembly in such a manner as to maintain the sterility of the needle until needed for performing the venipuncture.

Procedure

1. Make certain you have accurately identified the patient. For hospital patients, this may be done by checking the wrist band on the patient's arm. Never rely on the statement of a bedfast patient to obtain the

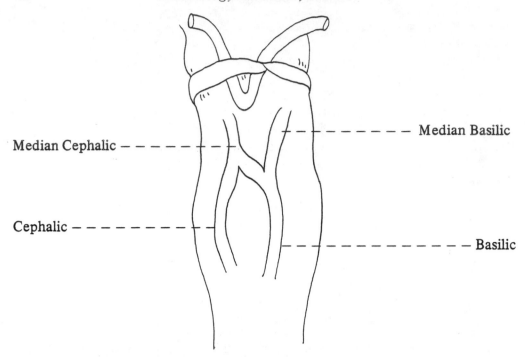

Median Cephalic – – – – – – – – – – –

Median Basilic

Cephalic – – – – – – – – – –

Basilic

Figure 4. Veins of forearm with point of application of the tourniquet. Redrawn from Barbara A. Brown: *Hematology, Principles and Procedures,* 2nd ed., 1976. Courtesy of Lea & Febiger, Philadelphia, Pennsylvania.

correct name! Compare the information on the requisition form with that on the wrist band to assure that you have the correct patient. When collecting from an outpatient, ask for his/her name. A mislabeled tube of blood for type and crossmatch can lead to a patient's death.

2. Assemble the equipment to be used.
3. Apply the tourniquet several inches above the puncture site as shown in Figure 4, just tightly enough to compress the tissues of the arm.
4. Ask the patient to make a tight fist. This makes the veins more easily palpable.
5. Select a suitable vein for puncture by palpating the area with your index finger. Choose a vein that is well anchored in tissue so it will not roll when the needle is first inserted. Palpation will enable you to find veins that are not easily visible. The veins will feel similar to an elastic tube. Trace the path of the vein chosen for puncture.
6. Cleanse the area with the alcohol swab.
7. Grasp the patient's arm just below the puncture site, pulling the skin tightly downward with your thumb.
8. Hold the vacuum system (or syringe) with the opposite hand between the thumb and the last three fingers.
9. The needle should be placed in the same direction the vein is running. Hold the syringe or vacuum system at a 15 degree angle with the patient's arm, bevel up.
10. The vein should be entered slightly below the area where it can be seen,

slightly to the side where more tissue is present to serve as an anchor for the needle and to prevent seepage of blood along the backside of the needle. Never attempt to enter the vein at a right angle.

11. The blood will begin to flow into the syringe, if used. Do not pull back the plunger too hard during collection as this may cause the blood to hemolyze, the vein to collapse, or inadvertently pull the needle out of the vein.

12. If the vacuum system is used, as soon as the needle is in the vein, push the vacuum tube in as far as it will go. Be careful that you keep the needle steady as you may inadvertently push it through the vein.

13. The tourniquet may be released as soon as the blood enters the tube or it may be left on until the process is complete. When collecting multiple samples, however, the tourniquet should be released to allow adequate blood flow. The patient may open his/her fist as soon as the blood begins to flow.

14. Release the tourniquet before the needle is removed from the vein.

15. Apply a clean, dry gauze pad to the site and gently withdraw the needle, applying a little pressure as withdrawal is made.

16. Immediately apply pressure to the point of puncture and maintain pressure for several minutes until bleeding has stopped. The patient may keep the arm straight and elevate it above the heart.

17. Disposable needles and syringes are appropriately discarded.

18. The specimens are appropriately labeled (patient name, hospital number, date, and time drawn). This must be done before you leave the patient or proceed to collect blood from another patient. Specimens may be appropriately labeled prior to the venipuncture if desired. *It is extremely important, however, that all samples are properly and positively identified.*

19. Be very careful not to stick yourself with the patient's needle. If this happens, report it to your supervisor as soon as possible on the day of the accident.

20. Check the patient's wound to make certain that bleeding has ceased.

Discussion

Sometimes the blood will "seep" into the surrounding tissues and leave a swollen, black and blue area known as a *hematoma*. A hematoma may be caused by:

1. failure to have the needle completely in the vein;
2. completely puncturing the vein by going through it;
3. failure to release the tourniquet before withdrawing the needle;
4. failure to apply pressure quickly enough or for a sufficient length of time;
5. repeated puncture of the vein.

Care must be taken to avoid these poor techniques during venipuncture.

SAMPLE PREPARATION

Analyses are performed on plasma, whole blood, or serum. If plasma or whole blood is to be used, it is necessary to add substances to the sample to prevent clotting. These substances are called anticoagulants. Their modes of action to prevent coagulation are somewhat different.

Anticoagulants Commonly Used for Hematology Procedures

Heparin

0.1 to 0.2 mg of saturated heparin per 1.0 ml of whole blood is used. Coagulation is prevented for approximately 24 hours. Heparin combines with antithrombin III to inhibit thrombin from acting upon fibrinogen. Heparinized blood smears have a blue background when stained with Wrights' stain and are unsatisfactory for blood smear morphologic examination. Heparin causes very little shrinkage of erythrocytes and is a good anticoagulant for the prevention of hemolysis.

Ammonium Oxalate and Potassium Oxalate

A mixture of these two substances, sometimes called double oxalate or balanced oxalate, consists of six parts of ammonium oxalate and four parts of potassium oxalate; 2 mg per 1 ml of whole blood is used. The mixture prevents coagulation by binding and precipitating calcium in the blood. The double oxalate is not generally used in routine hematology because it causes crenation of erythrocytes, vacuoles in granulocytes, and morphological alterations in lymphocytes and monocytes.

Trisodium Citrate

Trisodium citrate is one of the anticoagulants of choice for coagulation studies, depending upon the reagents used in the test procedures. It is also used in the collection of blood for transfusions. One part of a 3.8% aqueous solution of sodium citrate is used to nine parts of whole blood in coagulation studies. It prevents coagulation by binding calcium in a soluble complex.

Sodium Oxalate

A second type of anticoagulant used in coagulation studies is sodium oxalate. It is used in a concentration of one part 0.1M sodium oxalate to nine parts of whole blood. The sodium oxalate combines with calcium to form insoluble calcium oxalate and thus prevents coagulation.

EDTA (versene or sequestrene)

EDTA is the disodium or dipotassium salt of ethylene diaminetetraacetic acid. It is the most widely used anticoagulant for hematological studies. The potassium salt is more soluble than the sodium salt. 1.2 mg per 1 ml of blood is used. It removes calcium from the blood in the prevention of coagulation. The integrity of cell morphology is maintained for many hours and may be used for the preparation of blood smears up to two hours after collection. Blood may be stored in EDTA at 4°C for 24 hours without any effect shown in the hemoglobin, hematocrit, leukocyte count, or erythrocyte count. EDTA is an excellent anticoagulant for the prevention of platelet clumping.

When blood is added to the tube containing the anticoagulant, adequate mixing is necessary regardless of whether a liquid or dry anticoagulant is used. Inadequate mixing can result in the formation of small clots, which would necessitate obtaining a new specimen.

STUDY QUESTIONS

1. Why is it necessary that some equipment be kept in the storage cabinet areas?
2. What are the two types of glassware used in the clinical laboratory?
3. Which type of glassware is reusable?
4. Why is the proper cleaning of glassware so important?
5. What is the average adult blood volume?
6. Normal blood contains approximately _____ percent of plasma.
7. True or false: The X designation on the microscope eyepiece or objective indicates the number of times the object is magnified.
8. The 40X objective is used for _____ procedure.
9. The 10X objective is used for _____ procedure.
10. The 100X objective is used for _____ .
11. Why is immersion oil used in microscopy?
12. Define numerical aperture.
13. What precautions must be taken to keep the microscope clean?
14. Briefly outline the steps in obtaining blood from a fingertip puncture.
15. What is the size range of the needles used in routine venipunctures?
16. True or false: During venipuncture the tourniquet must be released as soon as the needle is in the vein.
17. Briefly outline the procedure for doing a venipuncture.
18. Define hematoma.
19. List some causes of hematomas.
20. Which anticoagulant does not bind with calcium to prevent coagulation of blood?
21. What is the difference between plasma and serum?
22. Which anticoagulant is the anticoagulant of choice for routine hematological studies?
23. Which anticoagulants are generally used for most coagulation studies?
24. Describe the proper use of:
    a. a To Deliver, blow-out pipet
    b. a To Deliver, drain-out pipet
    c. a To Contain pipet

Chapter 2

LEUKOCYTE AND ERYTHROCYTE COUNTING PROCEDURES

OBJECTIVES

The student will learn the following:

1. parameters of a complete blood count (CBC).
2. the normal leukocyte values for men, women, children, and newborns.
3. diluents that may be used for performing hemocytometer white cell counts.
4. the procedure for performing and calculating hemocytometer white blood cell counts.
5. the sources of error in performing hemocytometer white cell counts.
6. diseases in which the white cell count may be increased.
7. diseases in which the white cell may be decreased.
8. the normal erythrocyte values for men, women, children, and newborns.
9. the diluents that may be used for performing hemocytometer red cell counts.
10. the procedure for performing and calculating hemocytometer red cell counts.
11. the sources of error in performing hemocytometer red cell counts.
12. diseases and/or conditions in which the red cell count may be increased.
13. diseases and/or conditions in which the red cell count may be decreased.

THE COMPLETE BLOOD COUNT (CBC)

In most clinical laboratories the complete blood count, which is commonly called a CBC, consists of a determination of the number of erythrocytes and leukocytes, a hemoglobin determination, hematocrit determination, a differential leukocyte count, an examination of the blood smear morphology, and the calculation of the red blood cell indices. The importance of the CBC cannot be underestimated. As a screening procedure, it is useful in the diagnosis of many diseases; it may indicate the ability of the individual to respond to certain diseases; it may be used to reflect the individual's progress in disease states.

Today most laboratories perform the routine CBC by using some type of automated or semiautomated instrument or instruments. The automated procedures will be discussed in a subsequent section. This section will be confined to the discussion and performance of the leukocyte and erythrocyte counts using a counting chamber (hemocytometer) with the manual technique.

LEUKOCYTE (WHITE BLOOD CELL) COUNT

The white cell count (WBC) is expressed as the number of white cells in 1 microliter of whole blood, The International Committee for Standardization in Hematology has now recommended that all units of volume be expressed in liters. Since 1 mm³ equals 1.00003 μl, an insignificant difference, the microliter will be used as equivalent to and in preference to cubic millimeter in this chapter. In a normal healthy individual, the white count will range between 4,500 and 10,000 white cells per microliter of blood. This will vary with age, time of day, amount of exercise, time of last meal, etc.

Increased counts (leukocytosis) may be seen in—
    bacterial infections
    appendicitis
    leukemia
    hemolytic disease of the newborn
    pregnancy
    uremia
    ulcers
    normal newborn
Decreased counts (leukopenia) may be seen in—
    measles
    typhoid fever
    infectious hepatitis
    rheumatoid arthritis
    cirrhosis of the liver
    influenza
    other viral diseases
    radiation therapy
    drug therapy

Manual White Blood Count (WBC)

The procedure for performing a hemocytometer WBC count will be given in detail. The procedures outlined will be the same as those for the red cell count and platelet count; they will be presented only once. Familiarize yourself with these procedures before attempting to perform either type of count. It will take many attempts before these techniques will be mastered. Manipulation of pipets, counting chambers, cover slips, and other small equipment necessitates much patience and practice in order to become precise and accurate in making dilutions and performing the counts.

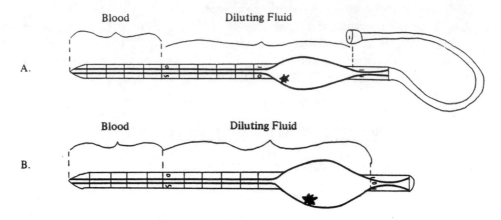

Figure 5. (A) White cell pipet with aspirator.
(B) Red cell pipet.

Except for platelet counts, hemocytometer methods are obsolete for routine blood cell counting in any but the smallest laboratories. However, it is still necessary for the technologist to be able to use this method effectively and to know its limitations.

Equipment and Reagents

1. white cell pipet and aspirator (Figure 5)
2. white cell diluting fluid (one of the following)
   a. 1% hydrochloric acid
   b. 2% acetic acid
   c. Turk's solution

glacial acetic acid	3 ml
1% aqueous gentian violet	1 ml
distilled water	100 ml
3. Kimwipes®
4. microscope
5. hemocytometer, or counting chamber, with cover glass (Figure 6)

Principle

Whole blood is mixed with a weak acid solution in order to dilute the blood and hemolyze the red cells. The weak acid does not destroy the nucleated cells; therefore, the white cells (and nucleated red cells) remain.

Dilution Procedure

1. The aspirator is placed on the pipet.
2. The well-mixed antiocoagulated blood is drawn to slightly above the 0.5 mark of the pipet.
3. Excess blood is wiped from the outside of the pipet.
4. With the index finger, retract the blood to exactly 0.5 mark.
5. Holding the pipet almost vertically, place the tip into the diluting

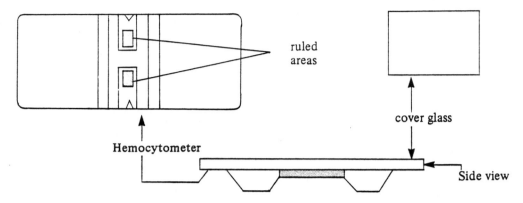

Figure 6. Hemocytometer and cover glass.

fluid and begin to draw the fluid into the pipet slowly, while gently rotating the pipet with your hand to ensure proper mixing. Aspirate the fluid until you reach the 11 mark. Repeat the procedure using a clean pipet if blood falls below the 0.5 mark, if the diluting fluid is aspirated too far above the 11 mark, or if air bubbles are present in the pipet. Fresh diluting fluid must be obtained if any blood has dropped into the vial, contaminating the fluid. Holding the pipet in a vertical position while aspirating the diluting fluid will help in eliminating air bubbles. If the level of diluting fluid goes only slightly above or slightly below the 11 mark, this is permissible and the dilution need not be repeated. A properly executed white cell dilution is 1 to 20 and, therefore, the dilution factor is 20.

6. Place the pipet in a horizontal position and firmly hold the index finger over the tip of the pipet before detaching the aspirator from the other end of the tube.

7. Two dilutions of the same specimen should be made.

Counting Procedures

1. Using a clean counting chamber and cover glass, carefully place the cover glass on top of the ruled area of the counting chamber.

2. Mix the diluted blood for approximately three minutes to ensure hemolysis of the red cells and adequate mixing. This may be done by placing the middle finger over one end of the pipet and the thumb over the other end and mixing by rotation of the hand back and forth. A mechanical shaker may also be used.

3. Filling the chamber:
   a. Hold the pipet in a vertical position with the index finger over the top of the pipet. Discard the first 4-5 drops of the dilution onto a Kimwipe.
   b. Remove excess fluid from the outside of the pipet. Be careful not to withdraw additional fluid out of the pipet with the Kimwipe.
   c. Place the tip of the pipet at the edge of the ruled area of the counting chamber, using the index finger to control the rate of the flow. Allow the dilution to creep under the cover glass until just

the ruled area is filled. Be careful not to move the cover glass or to flood the chamber. Steps 3a, 3b, and 3c must be done quickly so that the cells do not settle out. If the chamber has been improperly filled, reclean the chamber and cover glass. If enough dilution remains, remix, expel 2-3 drops and refill the chamber. Otherwise, a new dilution must be made.

   d. Fill the opposite side of the chamber with the second white count dilution.

   e. When both sides are filled, be careful not to jar the chamber or move the cover glass.

4. Counting the white blood cells.

   a. Carefully place the filled chamber on the microscope stage.

   b. Using low power (10X), and making the proper illumination adjustments, locate the ruled area of the chamber.

   c. Find one of the "W" squares on the chamber (Figure 7). For adequate counts, there should be even distribution of the cells in the "W" areas, with no more than a 12-cell variation between the four squares.

   d. Beginning with the upper left square, count all white cells in the four large "W" squares and add the results together to obtain the total counted. Count those cells touching the outside lines to the left and top of the large "W" squares, disregarding those that touch the right and lower outside margins (Figure 8).

   e. Count the cells on the opposite side of the chamber.

5. Calculating the white cell count.

   a. For each of the two counts performed, calculate the number of white blood cells per microliter of undiluted blood. Since the blood was diluted and the cells were counted in a volume less than 1 microliter, the number of cells counted must be multiplied by 2 correction factors:

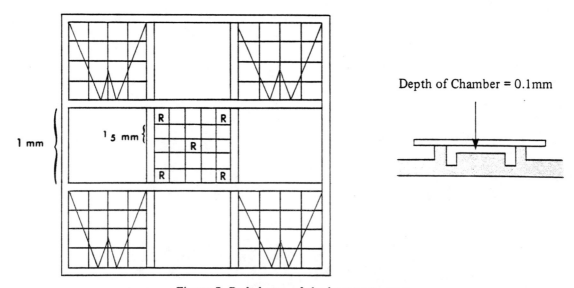

Figure 7. Ruled area of the hemocytometer.

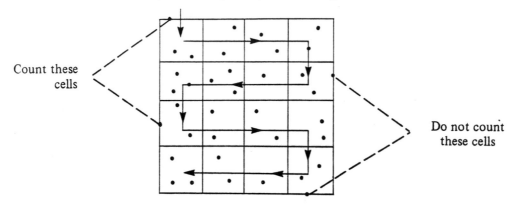

Figure 8. Counting cells in the "W" square.

(1) *dilution correction factor:* the blood was diluted 20 times in the pipet; therefore, the white cell dilution correction factor is 20.

(2) *volume correction factor:* the volume correction factor is 2.5, which was the volume in which the cells were counted.

$$\frac{volume\ correction}{factor} = \frac{volume\ in\ which\ white\ cells\ are\ reported}{volume\ in\ which\ white\ cells\ are\ counted} = \frac{1.0\ \mu l}{0.4\ \mu l} = 2.5$$

b. when the total number of cells in the 4 "W" sections are multiplied by the 2 correction factors, the WBC per microliter of blood is obtained.

$$number\ of\ white\ cells\ counted\ in\ 4W\ sections \times \frac{dilution}{correction\ factor} \times \frac{volume}{correction\ factor} = \frac{number\ of\ WBC}{in\ 1\ \mu l\ of\ whole\ blood}$$

Example: 100 × 20 × 2.5 = 5,000 WBC/μl
(5.0 × 10⁹/l)

Discussion

1. In certain conditions, the white count dilution preparation must be altered.

   a. If the white count is extremely high (above 25,000/μl), as in leukemia, it is advisable to use a red cell diluting pipet and make a 1:100 dilution or a 1:200 dilution. The procedure for the white count would proceed as described, but the volume correction factor would need to be altered accordingly.

   b. If the white count is below 2000 per μl, a smaller dilution should be used in order to achieve a more accurate count. For the procedure, the blood would be drawn to the 1.0 mark in the WBC pipet and diluted to the 11 mark to yield a 1:10 dilution. Counting would proceed as usual, but the dilution correction factor would change to 1:10 in this case.

2. The diluting fluid must be free from contamination by even small amounts of blood as this will alter the correct count.
3. The hemocytometer and cover glass must be clean and free of lint.
4. Pipets must be clean and dry. Dirty pipets will alter the proper dilution. Wet pipets will cause hemolysis of blood cells.
5. Correction of the white count is necessary if 5 or more nucleated red cells are present on the stained blood smear per 100 white cells.

$$\frac{corrected\ white}{cell\ count} = \frac{uncorrected\ white\ cell\ count \times 100}{100 + number\ of\ nucleated\ red\ cells\ per\ 100\ white\ cells}$$

6. Care must be taken when filling the hemocytometer to prevent overflowing of the ruled areas.
7. Delay in counting after the hemocytometer has been filled will result in inaccurate counts. If too much time has elapsed, the fluid will evaporate, causing the inaccuracy.
8. The margin of error of hemocytometer white counts falls within ±10%.

ERYTHROCYTE (RED BLOOD CELL) COUNT

The red blood cell count (RBC) is expressed as the number of red blood cells in 1 microliter of whole blood. The normal values for the red cell count will vary depending upon the sex and age of the individual. The average normal values follow.

Females: 3.6-5.5 million per μl
Males: 4.5-6.0 million per μl
Newborn: 5.0-6.5 million per μl

During childhood and adolescence the normal values for the red cell count will be slightly below the normal adult values. As with the white cell count, there are two methods for counting red blood cells: the automated (or semiautomated) methods and the hemocytometer method. The hemocytometer method is very similar to the white counting procedure. The hemocytometer procedure will not be presented in detail as it has been previously presented. The automated procedure will be presented in a subsequent section.

Increased counts (erythrocytosis) may be seen in—
    polycythemia vera
    dehydration
    hemoconcentration
    pulmonary disease
    heart disease
    hemoglobinopathies
    newborn
    stress
Decreased counts (anemia) may be seen in—
    bone marrow failure syndromes
    hemolytic disorders
    hemoglobinopathies
    vitamin B_{12} deficiency
    iron deficiency

enzyme deficiencies
intrinsic red cell defects
folate deficiency

Equipment and Reagents

1. red cell pipets and aspirator (Figure 5)
2. red cell diluting fluid. The red cell diluting fluids are isotonic to the red cells to prevent hemolysis or crenation. White cells are also preserved. Any one of the following diluting fluids may be used:
   a. Hayem's solution
   b. Gower's solution
   c. Sodium chloride (0.85% w/v)
3. Kimwipes
4. microscope
5. hemocytometer and cover glass (Figure 6). Referring to Figure 7, note the "R" squares shown. These are the areas to be counted for the red cell count. Each "R" area represents 0.04 mm. The chamber depth is 0.1 mm. The total volume held in the 5 "R" squares is 0.02 μl.

Principle

Whole blood is diluted with an isotonic diluting fluid to facilitate counting and prevent hemolysis of the red blood cells. A few white cells may also be present in the dilution. During the counting procedure white cells may be mistakenly counted as red cells, but the numbers are insignificant in the final red cell count. (In a 1:200 dilution, the number of white cells will be very small.)

Procedure

1. The aspirator is placed on the red cell pipet.
2. The well-mixed blood is drawn to the 0.5 mark, excess blood is removed from the exterior of the pipet, and dilution to the 101 mark is made. This gives a 1:200 dilution. A second dilution is made on the same specimen.
3. The dilution is shaken for three minutes (or 1 minute with the Yankee Pipet Shaker).
4. A clean hemocytometer is filled using both pipets (one dilution filling each side of the hemocytometer). Five or six drops of the dilution are expelled prior to filling the chambers. Allow the red cells to settle in the chamber for approximately 2-3 minutes before counting.
5. Counting the red cells.
   a. Place the hemocytometer carefully on the microscope stage.
   b. Using low power (10X), locate the large center square in the middle of the ruled area. Check for even distribution of the cells.
   c. Rotate the objective head to the 40X objective.
   d. Move the counting chamber and locate the upper corner "R" square (sub-divided into 16 smaller squares).
   e. Count all cells in the "R" square; move the chamber to the other

"R" squares and complete the counting of these areas. If there is a variation of more than 20 cells from one "R" square to another, distribution is not good and you must reshake the pipet, discard the first 4 drops, and refill a clean chamber. Repeat the count. Remember to count the cells on two of the outer margins but exclude those lying on the other two exterior lines.

6. Calculating the red cell count.

a. For each of the two counts performed, calculate the number of red blood cells per microliter of undiluted blood. Since the blood is diluted 1:200 and the cells are counted in a volume less than 1 microliter, the number of cells counted must be multiplied by 2 correction factors:

(1) *dilution correction factor:* the blood is diluted 200 times in the pipet, therefore, the red cell dilution correction factor is 200.

(2) *volume correction factor:* the volume correction factor is 50, which is the volume in which the cells are counted:

$$\frac{volume\ correction}{factor} = \frac{volume\ in\ which\ red\ cells\ are\ reported}{volume\ in\ which\ red\ cells\ are\ counted} = \frac{1.0\ \mu l}{0.02\ \mu l} = 50$$

b. when the total number of cells in the 5 "R" sections is multiplied by 2 correction factors, the RBC per microliter of blood is obtained.

$$\frac{number\ of\ red\ cells}{counted\ in\ 5R\ squares} \times \frac{dilution}{correction\ factor} \times \frac{volume}{correction\ factor} = \frac{number\ of\ RBC}{in\ 1\ \mu l\ of\ whole\ blood}$$

Example: $\quad 500 \quad \times \quad 200 \quad \times \quad 50 \quad = \quad 5,000,000/\mu l$
$(5.0 \times 10^{12}/l)$

Discussion

1. In conditions where the red count is very high, as in polycythemia, dehydration, or conditions of hemoconcentration, a larger dilution should be made to give a more accurate count. Draw the blood to the 0.3 mark and dilute to 101, giving a dilution factor of 333.

2. Extremely low red counts should be done using smaller dilutions. Draw the blood to the 1.0 mark in the pipet and dilute to 101, giving a dilution factor of 100.

3. The diluting fluid should be free from contamination.

4. All equipment must be free from dirt and dust and should be completely dry.

5. Do not allow evaporation of the fluid as this will cause inaccurate counts.

6. If the red cells are agglutinated when using Hayem's diluting fluid, the dilution should be repeated using Gower's solution or saline as the diluting fluid. Conditions of hyperglobulinemia will sometimes cause

rouleau formation or clumping of the red cells when Hayem's solution is used.

7. The range of error for a manual red count will usually be approximately ±20% with minimum error being ±10% and maximum error being ±30%.

Sources of Error in Hemocytometer Red and White Cell Counts

There are many sources of error in manual cell counting procedures, which contribute to inaccurate values. Some of these are listed below.

1. Failure to have blood exactly on the 0.5 mark of the pipet.
2. Failure to dilute the cells accurately to the 11 or 101 mark of the pipet.
3. Failure to shake or mix the dilution adequately.
4. Failure to discard the first 4-5 drops of dilution before filling the chamber. The dilution factor is created between the 1.0 mark and the 11 and 101 marks of the pipets. The stem of the pipet, therefore, contains only diluting fluid, which must be discarded.
5. Failure to fill the counting chamber properly—overflowing or air bubbles in the chamber.
6. Touching the cover glass with the fingers or microscope objective.
7. Using dirty, greasy, or wet equipment.
8. Failure to wipe excess blood from exterior of the pipet, thus contaminating the diluting fluid.
9. Using broken pipets: broken pipet tips will alter the dilution factor.
10. Mistakes in counting, calculation, or handling of the specimen.

QUALITY CONTROL IN THE HEMOCYTOMETER METHOD

When performing hemocytometer cell counts, the accuracy of the results is susceptible to a large margin of error. The minimum range of error in hemocytometer counting is usually about ±10%. Errors may result from a variety of causes: methods of sampling, technical errors, personnel errors, or improper preservation of the sample. It is important that some measure of the control of accuracy be made.

Reference controls may be purchased to use to monitor the degree of accuracy in performing all laboratory analyses. Normal and abnormal controls, which have assayed values, must be used to monitor laboratory accuracy and/or precision.

Hematology reference cells are used in conjunction with the unknowns to assess the degree of the accuracy of the test results. A red cell count and a white cell count of the reference cells must be performed as a routine part of the hemocytometer counting procedures. These cells are handled in the same manner as the unknown samples. See Chapter 10 for a more detailed discussion of quality control.

STUDY QUESTIONS

1. List the parameters of a complete blood count.
2. List the normal values for the following:
   a. erythrocyte count _____

　　b. leukocyte count _____

3. When the hemocytometer is to be used for cell counting, the dilution of the blood used to count the white blood cells is _____.

4. The usual dilution for counting red cells by hemocytometry is _____

5. The size of each "W" section of the hemocytometer is _____.

6. What is the depth of a hemocytometer when it is filled?

7. What physical property of the white cell diluting fluid is necessary to give accurate results?

8. List three solutions that are used as white cell diluents.

9. What physical property of the red cell diluting fluid is of utmost importance in maintaining the cellular integrity?

10. List three solutions that may be used for red cell dilutions.

11. What is the area of each "R" square of the hemocytometer?

12. What is the significance of the number of white cells in the red cell dilution?

13. What are the formulas for computing the red and white blood cell counts using hemocytometry?

14. 50, 40, 80, 86, and 38 red cells were counted in the 5 "R" squares. What is the value of this count?

15. What is the formula for correcting a white cell count for the presence of nucleated red cells?

16. Define:
　　a. leukocytopenia
　　b. erythrocytosis

17. List two conditions in which there is an increase in the number of red blood cells.

18. Why are the first 4-5 drops of fluid eliminated from the red and white cell pipets before filling the hemocytometer?

19. The microscope objective used to count white cells is _____

20. The microscope objective used to count red cells is _____

Chapter 3

HEMATOCRIT DETERMINATION, HEMOGLOBINOMETRY, AND RED CELL INDICES

OBJECTIVES

The student will learn and define the following:

1. hematocrit.
2. the normal hematocrit values for men, women, newborns, and young children.
3. the procedures for performing the hematocrit determination.
4. the conditions with which high or low hematocrit values may be associated.
5. the functions of hemoglobin.
6. the normal hemoglobin values for men, women, children, and the newborn.
7. the procedure for establishing a hemoglobin standard curve (cyanmethemoglobin method).
8. the reactions that occur when cyanmethemoglobin reagent is added to the blood.
9. the procedures for determining the hemoglobin value of a blood sample.
10. the forms of hemoglobin that are measured at a wavelength of 540 nm.
11. the sources of error in performing the procedure for determining the hemoglobin value.
12. the conditions in which high or low hemoglobin values may be associated.
13. MCV, MCH, MCHC.
14. the normal values for MCH, MCV, MCHC.
15. calculation of the MCV, MCH, MCHC given the values of the erythrocyte count, hematocrit, and/or hemoglobin.
16. the diagnostic significance of the mean corpuscular values.

THE HEMATOCRIT OR PACKED RED CELL VOLUME

The hematocrit is the volume of packed erythrocytes expressed as a percentage of the volume of whole blood in a sample. When anticoagulated whole blood is centrifuged, the space occupied by the packed red cells is called the hematocrit value. Due to the simplicity of the procedure and the reproducibility of the results, it is one of the more accurate laboratory tests. Hematocrit values will closely parallel the hemoglobin and red blood cell

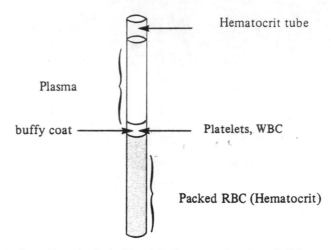

Figure 9. Centrifuged whole blood in hematocrit tube. (Cell layers shown.)

values. The venous hematocrit may be slightly higher than the hematocrit obtained from a capillary skin puncture.

During centrifugation the heavier particles fall to the bottom of the tube, while lighter particles will settle on top of the heavier ones, as shown in Figure 9.

The reading is made at the top of the red blood cell layer.

The normal values for the hematocrit will vary with the sex and age of the individual. Altitude also has an effect, in that individuals who live in high altitudes have higher hematocrits than those living at sea level. Average normal values follow:

Females:	37%-47%
Males:	47%-54%
Newborns:	50%-62%

Children and adolescents tend to have slightly lower values than adults.

High values may be seen in polycythemia (primary or secondary), in dehydration, and hemoconcentration. Low hematocrit values may be associated with the following conditions:

anemia

leukemia

hemodilution due to excessive fluid infiltration of the blood

The two manual methods for determining the hematocrit are the micro method and the macro method. The micro method is generally the method of choice in today's laboratory. The hematocrit may be computed by some of the automated instruments currently being used and, when used, is the method of choice in laboratories using these instruments. Dried heparin, balanced oxalate, or EDTA are satisfactory anticoagulants for the collection of the sample.

Microhematocrit Method (Adams)

Only the micro method will be discussed in detail.

Equipment and Reagents

1. capillary tubes, approximately 7 cm × 1 mm

   a. plain tubes if anticoagulated blood is to be used

   b. heparinized tubes if capillary blood is to be used (1:1000 dilution, dried)

2. clay for sealing the tubes
3. microhematocrit centrifuge, capable of 10,000-12,000 G
4. microhematocrit reader or other method for measurement

Principle

Whole blood is centrifuged to pack the red blood cells. The volume occupied by the red blood cells is measured and expressed as a percent of the whole blood volume.

Procedure

1. Fill two capillary tubes to approximately three-quarters full with well-mixed blood. (Air bubbles will not affect the principle but denote poor technique and may shorten the length of the column of blood.)
2. Seal one end with clay. (A hot flame may be used to seal the tube also.)
3. Place the tubes in the grooves of the centrifuge head opposite each other, with the sealed end away from the center of centrifuge and against the rubber gasket.
4. Centrifuge for 5 minutes at 10,000-12,000 G. The centrifuge has no speed control and will operate at full speed and automatically shut off. (Some laboratories will vary centrifugation time.)
5. Remove the tubes and read the hematocrit values of both tubes. The values should agree within ±2%. If not, repeat the procedure. The value is read from the hematocrit reader in the following manner.
   a. The capillary tube is placed in the groove in the plastic holder, aligning the bottom of the packed red cells with the bottom edge of the reader bar. The bottom of the red cell column should be at 0.
   b. Move the plastic holder until the meniscus of the plasma in the tube coincides with the 100 mm mark on the reader.
   c. Read the hematocrit percentage from the reader line directly corresponding to the top line of the packed red cell column.
6. Report the percent of packed red blood cells.

Discussion

The hematocrit reflects the concentration of red cells, not the total red cell mass. The hematocrit is low in hydremia of pregnancy but the total number of erythrocytes is not reduced. The hematocrit may be normal, even high, in shock accompanied by hemoconcentration, although the total red cell mass may be considerably decreased due to blood loss. The hematocrit values are unreliable immediately following a loss of blood, even if moderate, and immediately following transfusions.

Macrohematocrit Method

The macrohematocrit method is similar to the microhematocrit method except that a larger tube, a Wintrobe tube, is used for the procedure, and the centrifugation time is altered.

The graduated tube is filled to the 0 (or 10) mark with well-mixed whole anticoagulated blood. The tube is centrifuged in a centrifuge with a bucket head for 30 minutes at 2500 RPM. The hematocrit value is read from the scale on the tube and calculated as follows:

$$hematocrit\ in\ \% = \frac{100 \times height\ of\ red\ blood\ cell\ column\ in\ mm}{height\ of\ whole\ blood\ specimen\ in\ mm}$$

This method is rarely used today because it is very time-consuming and it requires much more blood than the micro method. The normal values for this procedure are the same as for the microhematocrit method.

Sources of Error in Hematocrit (Micro and Macro Method)

1. Inadequate centrifugation: Centrifugation must be of adequate speed and duration of time. The red cells must be packed so that additional centrifugation will not reduce the volume any further. In general, the higher the hematocrit, the more powerful the centrifugal force required. During centrifugation leukocytes, platelets, and plasma are trapped between the red cells. Generally the number of leukocytes and platelets result in insignificant error. The amount of trapped plasma is somewhat greater than leukocytes or platelets, but this too produces little practical consequence unless insufficient centrifugal force is used in the procedure. The lower the centrifugal force (or shorter the centrifugal time), the larger the amount of trapped plasma. In high hematocrits, there is more plasma entrapment than in low hematocrits, and the amount of trapped plasma is larger with the macro method than the micro method.
2. If blood is over-oxalated, the hematocrit will be falsely low due to cell shrinkage. Heparin is the best anticoagulant to use because it causes the least shrinkage of all the anticoagulants. However, few laboratories use heparin for routine hematological studies. EDTA and oxalates do yield accurate values if the proper ratio of blood to anticoagulant is maintained.
3. Failure to seal the hematocrit tubes will result in low values due to the greater loss of red blood cells than of plasma.
4. Failure to mix the blood specimen thoroughly before using will result in the cells not being properly suspended.
5. Prolonged stasis caused by constriction of the arm with a tourniquet for one minute or longer will result in falsely high hematocrits of 2.5% to 5%.
6. A free flow of blood from a skin puncture for the micro method is essential. Interstitial fluids may dilute the total red cell mass resulting in falsely low hematocrit values.
7. With good technique, the accuracy of the hematocrit is ±1%.

HEMOGLOBINOMETRY

Hemoglobin is a pigmented substance within the red cells that has three functions: to carry oxygen from the lungs to tissues; to assist in the transportation of carbon dioxide from the tissues to the lungs; and to act as a blood buffer. Hemoglobinometry is the measurement of the concentration of hemoglobin in the blood. Anemia, a decrease below normal of the hemoglobin concentration, red cell count, or hematocrit, is a common condition and often a complication of other diseases. The correct determination of the hemoglobin value is important because anemia is frequently masked in many diseases by other manifestations.

The concentration of hemoglobin is expressed in grams per 100 milliliter of blood, or grams per deciliter (g/dl).

The normal value for hemoglobin will vary with the age and sex of the individual. Altitude also has an effect in that the normal hemoglobin concentration for residents at high altitudes is higher than for those living at sea level. Average normal values follow:

> Females: 14 g/dl ± 2 g/dl
> Males: 16 g/dl ±2 g/dl
> Newborn: 14-20 g/dl

Children to age 10 will be slightly lower than adults. During pregnancy, there is retention of body fluids, which results in increased plasma volume and the red cells become less concentrated (hemodilution). The hemoglobin levels are reduced as a result. The variations are referred to as physiological variations, i.e. variations due to age, sex, altitude, and pregnancy.

Hemoglobin values may drop below normal in many conditions such as—

> anemia (all types)
> leukemia
> multiple myeloma
> excessive radiation therapy
> excessive chemotherapy

Hemoglobin values may be high in dehydration, polycythemia (primary and secondary), and conditions of hemoconcentration.

The methods used in hemoglobinometry can be grouped into four main classes: colorimetric methods, gasometric methods, specific gravity methods, and chemical methods. In most procedures a measured amount of blood is pipetted into a given volume of diluting solution. The diluting solution functions to—

1. hemolyze the red cells
2. liberate the hemoglobin
3. stabilize the hemoglobin by converting it to some other form

Only one of the colorimetric methods will be discussed in detail in this manual. Direct matching and acid and alkali hematin methods, three older colorimetric methods, are not satisfactory for photometry and, therefore, are no longer used in routine hemoglobinometry. In these older procedures, the hemoglobin was often not stabilized and decomposition led to erroneous results. The cyanmethemoglobin method is most commonly used today. In this procedure, the stabilized hemoglobin colors the diluting solution. The depth of color is proportional to the concentration of the hemoglobin. The measurement is performed in an instrument called a colorimeter by comparing the unknown sample of hemoglobin to a standard or known amount of hemoglobin.

Photoelectric Colorimetric Methods

Photoelectric colorimetric methods are the methods of choice today. These methods involve the use of an electronic colorimeter, either a spectrophotometer, or a photometer (Figure 10).

Principles of Spectrophotometry

1. A wavelength selector filters out all but one wavelength of light from a white light source. This is called a wavelength of monochromatic light.
2. This wavelength of light passes through the solution containing the colored molecules that are to be measured. Some of the light is absorbed by the molecules in the solution and some light is transmitted, or passed through the solution.
3. The transmitted light strikes a photoelectric cell, which converts light energy to electrical energy. The photoelectric cell sends out an electric current that is proportional to the intensity of the transmitted light. The amount of electric current produced is measured and read out on a galvanometer whose scale is calibrated to read percentage of light transmitted.

The principle involved is known as Beer's Law or the Beer-Lambert Law. The more concentrated the sample molecules in the solution, the more light is absorbed and the less light is transmitted. The less concentrated the sample molecules in solution, the less light is absorbed, and the amount of light transmitted is therefore greater.

Colorimetric tests are valid only if color development is directly proportional to the concentration of the substance in the solution. Time for color development must be allowed before readings are taken.

In summary, the intensity of the beam of monochromatic light entering and leaving the solution depends on the concentration in the solution.

Cyanmethemoglobin Method

This method is the most widely used colorimetric method today.

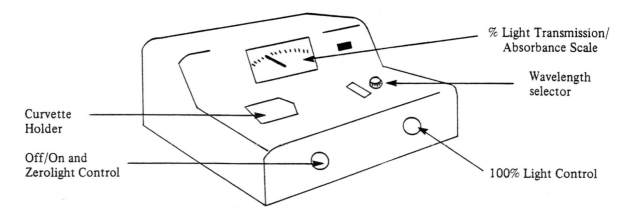

Figure 10. Bausch and Lomb® Spectronic "20"®.

Equipment and Reagents

1. Drabkin's reagent: This reagent is available commercially in liquid or dry pack. The liquid form is stable for one month if stored in a cool place in a brown bottle. Caution: it must be pipetted either with a rubber bulb attached to the pipet or by an autodilutor or from a burette, but *never by mouth*.
2. test tubes, 13 × 100 mm
3. Sahli pipets or disposable pipets, 0.02 ml
4. Kimwipes
5. colorimeter or spectrophotometer with matched cuvettes

Principle

Whole blood is added to the Drabkin's reagent, which contains potassium ferricyanide and potassium cyanide. The red blood cells are lysed and the hemoglobin released. The ferricyanide converts the hemoglobin iron from the ferrous state to the ferric state to form methemoglobin:

$$Hb(Fe^{++}) \xrightarrow[\left[K_3\,Fe\,(CN)_6\right]]{\substack{\text{potassium}\\\text{ferricyanide}}} Hb(Fe^{+++})$$

Methemoglobin then combines with potassium cyanide to form the stable pigment, cyanmethemoglobin, which can be measured colorimetrically:

$$Hb(Fe^{+++}) \xrightarrow[\text{(KCN)}]{\substack{\text{potassium}\\\text{cyanide}}} Hb(Fe^{+++})CN$$

The color intensity of this compound is measured at a wavelength of 540 nm. The optical density of the solution is proportional to the concentration of the hemoglobin. All forms of hemoglobin are measured with this method *except sulfhemoglobin*.

Procedure

1. Prepare a standard curve in the following manner:
   a. Mark a series of test tubes B (blank), 5, 10, 15, 20.
   b. Pipet the following volumes of cyanmethemoglobin standard and cyanmethemoglobin reagent (Drabkin's solution) into the correspondingly marked tubes and mix well:

Tube	Reagent	Standard	Concentration of Hemoglobin
B	6.0 ml	0.0 ml	0.0 g/dl
5	4.5 ml	1.5 ml	5.0 g/dl
10	3.0 ml	3.0 ml	10.0 g/dl
15	1.5 ml	4.5 ml	15.0 g/dl
20	0.0 ml	6.0 ml	20.0 g/dl

   c. Transfer the solutions to well-matched cuvettes and measure the percent transmittance (or the absorbance) of each dilution against the blank at 540 nm.

  d. Plot the percent transmittance of each dilution on semilogarithmic graph paper (or the absorbance on regular graph paper). Plot the concentration on the abscissa (horizontal axis) and the %T or absorbance on the ordinate (vertical axis). A line connecting the reading of tubes marked 5, 10, and 15 should pass through or very near zero. This will be a straight-line curve. This chart can then be used to facilitate reading the test results of the unknown hemoglobin concentration.

2. Pipet exactly 5.0 ml of cyanmethemoglobin reagent into each of two test tubes #1 and #2.
3. Add 0.02 ml of capillary, or well-mixed anticoagulated blood to the reagent in test tube #2. Rinse the pipet at least three times with the reagent to assure that all of the blood has been removed from the pipet. (The Sahli pipet is a *To Contain* pipet and therefore must be rinsed to obtain all its contents.)
4. Mix the previous solution well and allow to sit at room temperature for at least ten minutes to permit the formation of cyanmethemoglobin.
5. Transfer the mixture to a cuvette and the reagent to a matching cuvette and read in a colorimeter or spectrophotometer at a wavelength of 540 nm (or yellow-green filter) using the reagent in tube #1 to blank the machine (set percent transmittance at 100%).
6. Refer to the standard curve for the actual hemoglobin value in grams per deciliter.

Discussion

1. The cyanmethemoglobin reagent must be crystal clear as well as the unknown sample-reagent mixture before a reading is taken. Cloudiness may be the result of contamination of the reagent and, in this case, a new reagent solution must be obtained. Cloudiness of the reagent-sample mixture may result from very high white blood cell counts, from hemoglobin S and hemoglobin C, from abnormal plasma globulins, or from lipemic blood. Whatever the cause, the mixture must be clear prior to reading the hemoglobin. HbS or HbC blood should be diluted 1:1 with distilled water, read on the colorimeter, and the reading multiplied by 2. 0.1 g of potassium carbonate should be added to samples containing high levels of abnormal globulins.
2. Accurate pipetting is of utmost importance. Clean, dry pipets, test tubes, and cuvettes must be used.
3. The colorimeter or spectrophotometer must be turned on at least 15 minutes prior to reading any standard or hemoglobin values.
4. A new standard curve should be run whenever alterations, replacements, repairs, or relocations of the instrument occur.
5. The same instrument and filter or wavelength *must* be used for both standards and unknowns.
6. A new standard curve should be run whenever a new lot number of reagent is used. It is recommended by manufacturers of reagents that new standard curves be run weekly. The unused portion of the standard vial must always be discarded.

7. Hemoglobin controls should always be run on a daily basis or with each group of unknowns. A high, low, and normal control should be available for use. Technical and personnel errors will be picked up if the hemoglobin control values do not fall within ±2 standard deviations of the mean assay value on the package.

Sources of Error

Some of the possible errors have been listed under the discussion. Additional sources of error are listed below:
1. Improper venipuncture technique may produce hemoconcentration, which will make the hemoglobin value too high. Improper technique in capillary sampling may cause errors in either direction.
2. Depending upon the method used, only certain forms of hemoglobin are measured. The cyanmethemoglobin method measures reduced hemoglobin, (hemoglobin not combined with oxygen), oxyhemoglobin (hemoglobin combined with oxygen), carboxyhemoglobin (hemoglobin combined with carbon monoxide), and methemoglobin (oxidized hemoglobin). Only sulfhemoglobin (hemoglobin combined with sulfur) is not measured. This method, therefore, most closely determines the amount of physiologically active hemoglobin.
3. Inaccurate pipets or inaccurate use of the pipets. Volumetric pipets must be used to pipet the reagent and the hemoglobin standard. Care must be taken to rinse the Sahli pipets completely.
4. Unmatched cuvettes may result in significant error.
5. Improperly calibrated photometer or colorimeter.
6. Improper procedure or technique.

Automated Hemoglobinometry

Semiautomated and automated equipment are widely used and have the advantages of eliminating many of the human errors. Many types of instruments are available today that are capable of performing the complete blood count, including hemoglobin measurement. Most of these instruments employ a colorimetric method for determining the hemoglobin concentration. The cyanmethemoglobin method is still the method of choice even in complete automation.

The principle of automated hemoglobinometry involves a specific dilution of blood with Drabkin's reagent; cyanmethemoglobin is formed (as in manual procedures), and the color intensity is measured colorimetrically at 525-550 nm, depending upon the type of instrument used in the laboratory. The hemoglobin value in grams per deciliter of blood will be displayed by the instrument or printed out by the automatic printer. Values are very accurate if the instrument is properly calibrated.

RED BLOOD CELL INDICES

The red blood cell indices are used to define the size and hemoglobin content of the average red blood cell in a blood sample. They consist of the MCV (mean corpuscular volume), MCH (mean corpuscular hemoglobin), and the MCHC (mean corpuscular hemoglobin concentration). The red cell indices are used as an aid in differentiating anemias. When these values are used with an examination of the red blood cells on a stained blood smear, a clear picture of the red cell morphology may be determined. *It must be remembered that the indices give only an average value.* Indices are only useful if they are reasonably accurate, and this depends upon the accuracy of the measurements from which they are calculated.

Mean Corpuscular Volume (MCV)

The MCV is defined as the volume of the average red blood cell in a sample population. The measurement is in cubic microns or femtoliters.* One femtoliter $= 10^{15}$ liters $= 1 \ \mu m^3$. Normal values range from 80 to 98 fl. The MCV is computed from the hematocrit and red blood count as follows:

Example: *Hematocrit = 40% (or .40)*
             Red Blood Count = 4,500,000/μl (4.5 × 10⁶/μl, 1 μl = 10⁹ fl)

$$MCV = \frac{volume \ of \ red \ blood \ cells \ in \ fl \ per \ \mu l \ of \ blood}{number \ of \ red \ blood \ cells \ per \ \mu l \ of \ blood}$$

$$MCV = \frac{.40 \times 10^9 \ fl/\mu l}{4.5 \times 10^6/\mu l}$$

$$MCV = \frac{40 \times 10 \ fl}{4.5}$$

$$MCV = 88.8 \ fl$$

Therefore, the formula for computation of the MCV is:

$$MCV = \frac{hematocrit \times 10}{red \ blood \ count \ in \ millions} \ fl$$

Discussion

The MCV indicates whether the red blood cells are normocytic (normal cells), macrocytic (large cells), or microcytic (small cells). Values below 80 fl indicate that the red blood cells are microcytic. Values above 98 fl indicate that the red blood cells are macrocytic. If the MCV is within the normal range, the red blood cells are normocytic.

Mean Corpuscular Hemoglobin (MCH)

The MCH is defined as the weight of hemoglobin in the average red blood cell in a sample population. The measurement is in micro-micrograms or picograms. The range of normal values is 27-32 picograms (pg). The MCH is computed from the hemoglobin and the red blood count as follows:

---

*fl is a new symbol that replaces the measurement of cubic micrometers (μm^3), cubic microns (μ^3); a femtoliter.

$$MCH = \frac{weight\ of\ hemoglobin\ in\ 1\ \mu l\ of\ blood}{number\ of\ red\ blood\ cells\ in\ 1\ \mu l\ of\ blood}$$

The hemoglobin value (in g/dl) must first be converted to pg/μl.

$$1\ g = 10^{12}\ pg$$
$$1\ ml = 10^3\ \mu l$$

Thus the weight (in pg) of hemoglobin in 1 μl can be determined as follows:

$$weight\ of\ hemoglobin\ in\ 1\ \mu l\ of\ blood = \frac{hemoglobin \times 10^{12}\ pg}{100 \times 10^3/\mu l}$$

$$= hemoglobin \times 10^7\ pg/\mu l$$

Example: *Hemoglobin = 14g/dl*
red blood count = 5,000,000/μl

$$MCH = \frac{14 \times 10^7\ pg/\mu l}{5.0 \times 10^6/\mu l}$$

$$MCH = \frac{14 \times 10}{5.0}\ pg$$

$$MCH = 28\ pg$$

Therefore, the formula for the computation of the MCH is:

$$MCH = \frac{hemoglobin\ (in\ grams) \times 10}{red\ blood\ count\ in\ millions}\ pg$$

Discussion

The MCH indicates the amount of hemoglobin in the red blood cells. Values lower than 27 pg indicate that the red blood cells are hypochromic (under color, indicating lack of a normal amount of hemoglobin). Normal values indicate that the red cells are normochromic (normal color, normal amount of hemoglobin). An elevated MCH will occur in macrocytic anemias and in some cases of spherocytosis where "hyperchromia" (above normal color) may be present. Hyperchromia indicates only that the red cells appear darker in color (on stained smears) and does not indicate an increased amount of intracellular hemoglobin. Theoretically this state (hyperchromia) is physiologically impossible, as the amount of hemoglobin depends on cell size, and the hemoglobin usually saturates the cell to its full extent and not any more.

Mean Corpuscular Hemoglobin Concentration (MCHC)

The MCHC is defined as the ratio of the amount of hemoglobin to the volume in which it is contained. It gives the concentration of hemoglobin in the average red blood cell in a sample population. The measurement is in percent. Normal values range from 32% to 38%. The MCHC is computed from the hemoglobin and the hematocrit as follows:

$$MCHC \ = \ \frac{hemoglobin \ in \ g/dl \times 100}{hematocrit/dl}$$

Example: hemoglobin = 14g/dl
            hematocrit = 40%

$$MCHC \ = \ \frac{14g/dl \times 100\%}{40 \ volumes/dl}$$

$$MCHC \ = \ \frac{14 \times 100}{40}$$

$$MCHC \ = \ 35\%$$

Therefore, the formula for the computation of the MCHC is:

$$MCHC \ = \ \frac{hemoglobin \times 100}{hematocrit} \ \%$$

Discussion

The MCHC indicates whether the red blood cells are normochromic or hypochromic. A value below 32% indicates hypochromia. A normal MCHC indicates the red blood cells are normochromic. The MCHC cannot be elevated above normal values because hemoglobin saturation is limited by the size of the red cell. The larger the red cell, the more hemoglobin it can hold. This amount of hemoglobin is normal for this cell size but is greater than that for a red cell of normal size.

STUDY QUESTIONS

1. Define hematocrit.
2. Write the normal hematocrit values for the following:
   a. men _____
   b. women _____
   c. newborn _____
   d. young children _____
3. Outline the procedures for performing the hematocrit determination (micro and macro methods).
4. List two conditions in which high hematocrit values could be found.
5. List two conditions in which low hematocrit values could be found.
6. What are the chemical reactions that occur when Drabkin's solution (cyanmethemoglobin reagent) is added to whole blood?
7. The wavelength used for the spectrophotometric measurement of hemoglobin is _____.
8. What is the purpose of using a blank in spectrophotometry?
9. List the normal hemoglobin values for the following:
   a. men _____
   b. women _____
   c. newborn _____
   d. young children _____
10. List two conditions in which high hemoglobin values could be found.

11. List two conditions in which low hemoglobin values could be found.
12. List three functions of hemoglobin.
13. What solution should be used as the blank in the cyanmethemoglobin method of hemoglobin measurement? Why is this solution used as the blank?
14. Outline the procedure for establishing the hemoglobin standard curve.
15. What volume of blood and volume of diluent are used to determine the hemoglobin value of an unknown blood sample in the cyanmethemoglobin method?
16. Define:
    a. MCV
    b. MCH
    c. MCHC
17. List the normal values for:
    a. MCV
    b. MCH
    c. MCHC
18. Calculate the MCV, MCH and MCHC using the following parameters:

    RBC = 5,000,000/ μl
    Hematocrit = 45%
    Hemoglobin = 15 g/dl
19. What are the diagnostic values of the mean corpuscular indices?

Chapter 4

PREPARATION OF A BLOOD SMEAR AND BLOOD SMEAR EXAMINATION

OBJECTIVES

The student will:

1. describe the process of manually preparing a blood smear.
2. give the purposes of the blood smear examination.
3. learn the meaning of the following:
   a. anisocytosis
   b. poikilocytosis
   c. polychromia (polychromasia)
   d. hypochromia
   e. hyperchromia
   f. microcytes
   g. macrocytes
   h. normocytes
4. learn the size range for normal erythrocytes.
5. describe and identify the following:
   a. spherocytes
   b. codocytes
   c. schistocytes
   d. drepanocytes
   e. siderocytes
   f. burr cells
   g. crenated cells
   h. rouleau formation
6. describe the following erythrocyte inclusions and indicate the composition of the inclusion structure:
   a. basophilic stippling
   b. Heinz bodies
   c. Howell-Jolly bodies
   d. siderotic granules
7. identify pathological or physiological conditions in which the following may be found:
   a. schistocytes
   b. burr cells
   c. macrocytes

    d. hypochromia

    e. spherocytes

    f. rouleau formation

    g. elliptocytosis

8. learn the morphological aspects of platelets which are examined from the blood smear.
9. learn the proper pH of Wright's or Wright-Giemsa stains for optimum blood smear staining.
10. learn the properties of the Wright's or Wright-Giemsa stain that aid identification of the cytochemical properties of blood cells.
11. learn the proper fixative for fixing the blood film to the glass slide prior to staining.
12. learn the principle of operation of the Hema-Tek Slide Stainer.

THE BLOOD SMEAR

Examination of a stained blood smear is an important parameter of the complete blood count. Microscopic study of the morphology of blood cells depends a great deal upon the proper preparation and staining of the blood smear. There are two manual procedures for making blood smears: the cover glass method and the slide method. There are instruments available which prepare blood smears by centrifugal force. Only the manual procedure will be discussed in this section. Many pathologists and hematologists prefer a well-made cover glass smear or the spun smear, but the slide smear is most commonly used.

Slide Method

1. Obtain two perfectly clean glass slides, one spreader slide, and, if using anticoagulated blood, two applicator sticks or a plain hematocrit tube.
2. If using anticoagulated blood, hold the two applicator sticks together and dip them into the well-mixed blood sample (or fill a hematocrit tube with blood).
3. Place a small drop of blood at one end of a slide, directly in the middle of the slide.
4. If using blood from a finger or toe, etc., place a drop of blood on the slide as stated above, being careful not to touch the skin with the slide.
5. Place the slide on the table or counter top with the drop of blood on the right (if you are right handed).
6. Elevate the opposite end of the slide by placing your first two fingers under the slide. With the right hand, hold the spreader slide with the thumb on one edge and the four fingers on the other edge. Place the spreader slide in front of the drop of blood, holding it at approximately a 25 degree angle from the bottom slide (Figure 11). Pull the top slide back until its back side encounters the drop of blood. As soon as the spreader slide touches the blood, the blood will begin to spread along the back edge of the spreader slide. *Be very careful that no blood gets in front of the slide.*

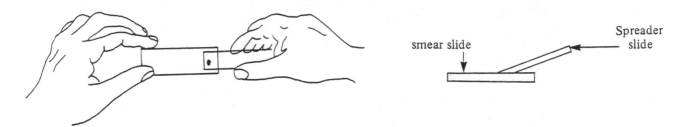

Figure 11. Method of holding slides for preparation of blood smear. Redrawn from Barbara A. Brown: *Hematology, Principles and Procedures*, 2nd ed., 1976. Courtesy of Lea & Febiger, Philadelphia, Pennsylvania.

7. Keeping the spreader slide at a 25 degree angle and pressed firmly against the bottom slide, push the spreader slide quickly and evenly to the other end of the bottom slide.
8. Prepare a second smear from the same specimen.
9. Allow the smears to air dry and label the thick end of the smear with the patient's name in pencil. If good smears have been made, they are now ready to be stained with Wright's stain or Wright-Giemsa stain.

Cover Slip Method

1. With the thumb and index finger of each hand, hold two cover slips by their edges.
2. Touch the center of one cover slip to a small drop of blood.
3. Gently place the second cover glass over the cover glass containing the blood (with drop of blood between the two slides), so that the two cover glasses form a 16-sided figure (Figure 12). As soon as the two cover glasses come together, the blood begins to spread between them. Just before the spreading is complete, evenly and smoothly, draw the cover glasses apart in a horizontal plane.
4. Allow the smears to air-dry and then stain with Wright's stain or Wright-Giemsa stain.

Criteria for a Good Blood Smear

1. The blood smear must gradually become thinner from the point of application.
2. The smear must have reasonable thickness and length.
3. The smear should not be wavy in appearance.
4. The end of the smear should be "feathered" and it should not extend to the end of the slide (Figure 13).
5. The smear must be smooth in appearance.

Discussion

1. All slides and cover glasses must be extremely clean.
2. If capillary blood is used, the smear must be made quickly. If the blood sits too long (beyond 3 seconds), coagulation will begin, platelets will

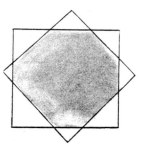

Figure 12. Cover glass method of making a blood smear. Redrawn from Barbara A. Brown: *Hematology, Principles and Procedures*, 2nd ed., 1976. Courtesy of Lea & Febiger, Philadelphia, Pennsylvania.

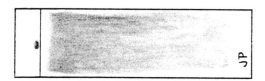

Figure 13. Blood smear with feathered edge.

form aggregates, and red cells and white cells will also appear clumped.

3. The size of the drop of blood used is very important. Too large a drop will result in smears too thick for accurate study. Too small a drop will result in smears too thin and too small for accurate study.
4. The spreader slide must be kept free of any blood on its front side prior to pushing it across the bottom slide.
5. The spreader slide should be kept firmly placed on the smear slide during the spreading process. Failure to do this will result in thick streaks in the smear.
6. The spreader slide must have a smooth, unbroken edge.

STAINING THE BLOOD SMEAR

Blood smears should be stained within two hours for best results. Two types of stains are normally used: Wright's stain and Wright-Giemsa stain. Wright's stain is more widely used in today's laboratory.

The examination of the cells of the blood is facilitated by staining the smear. In this way, the various cells become easily differentiated and the morphology more easily distinguished.

Principle

Wright's stain is a polychromatic stain, meaning the dyes present in the stain will produce multiple colors when the stain is added to cells. Wright's stain is a mixture of eosin and methylene blue. In Wright's stain the methylene blue is polychromed by heating or aging. Eosin is then added to the polychromed methylene blue and a precipitate is formed. The precipitate is then added to anhydrous, acetone-free methanol, yielding Wright's stain. The quantities of eosin and polychromed methylene blue must be very carefully controlled during the making of the Wright's stain powder in order to yield a neutral compound dye so that optimum staining results. In the staining process, when a buffer solution is added to the stain, ionization occurs, during which time the staining process takes place. Methylene blue ions are positively charged and stain acid components of the cells varying shades of blue to purple. The basic structures of the cell are stained orange to pink by the negatively charged, acid eosin ions. When both the basic and acid stains are taken up by the cytoplasmic or nuclear structures of the cell, a pink to lilac color develops, and the structures are called neutrophilic.

Equipment and Reagents (Manual Method)

1. Wright's stain or Wright-Giemsa stain
2. phosphate buffer (pH 6.4-6.8)
3. methyl alcohol (absolute, anhydrous, acetone-free)
4. staining rack

Manual Staining Procedures

1. Place slides on a staining rack, smear side up. Make sure the stain rack is level.
2. Fix the smears by flooding with methanol. This step is often omitted because fixation occurs by the methanol in the Wright's stain. If methanol is used, drain the excess methanol from the slides.
3. Flood the slides with Wright's stain. Set the timer for 3-4 minutes. When stain is first prepared, or first used, the staining time should be determined by trying several timings to determine the optimum time for best staining technique.
4. Add an equal amount of phosphate buffer to the stain on the slide, being careful not to remove any stain. Mix the two reagents on the slide by gently blowing back and forth over the solutions. If mixing is proper, a green metallic sheen will appear on the surface. Time for 5-7 minutes, depending on the procedure set for optimum staining.
5. Rinse the slide gently and thoroughly with tap water or distilled water.
6. Wipe the back of the slide to remove any stain.
7. Stand the slides on end to air dry. *Do not blot smears dry.*

Automated Procedure (Hema-Tek Slide Stainer)

1. The instrument is primed.
2. The dry blood smears are placed in the slots at the loading point facing left, with the feathered end away from you.
3. The smears advance into position face down on the staining plate.
4. Next, a switch activates the first pump, which delivers stain to the slides. The slides are stained by the stain that has spread between the metal plate and the surface of the smears.
5. The smears advance to the second positon and a second pump delivers the buffer to the smears. Stain and buffer mix as the smears advance.

6. Advance continues and a third pump delivers distilled water to rinse the slides.
7. The smears are dried by a current of warm air at the end of the plate. They are dropped off and stored in a collecting drawer. Twenty-five slides can be stained in approximately 30 minutes.

Discussion

1. During staining, the phosphate buffer controls the pH of the stain. If the pH is too acid, those cellular structures taking up the acid dye will stain well, while those structures that stain at a more alkaline pH will appear pale. For instance, cell nuclei and platelets prefer an alkaline pH while eosinophils and red blood cells take up an acid dye. In order to stain all cellular structures well, the pH of the phosphate buffer is critical.
2. Insufficint washing of the smears will result in precipitated stain remaining on the slide.
3. If the rinse water is left on the slides too long, or if the slides are excessively rinsed, the stain will fade.
4. New staining times may need to be established periodically due to the fact that the Wright's stain may change from standing.
5. Dry, stained cover glass smears are mounted, blood side down, on a slide, using a mounting medium.

EXAMINATION OF THE BLOOD SMEAR

An examination of the stained smear is performed for four purposes:
1. to examine the morphology of the red blood cells.
2. to examine the morphology of the platelets.
3. to give an estimate of platelet numbers (decreased, increased, normal).
4. to perform a differential white blood cell count.

Procedure for Examination of the Blood Smear

1. Locate the blood smear under low power and assess the general distribution of cells.
2. Select a thin, well-stained area where the erythrocytes just touch each other.
3. Add a drop of oil to the slide and switch to the oil immersion objective.
4. Count 100 consecutive leukocytes, identifying each by using a differential counter. (Chapter 5 will discuss the differential count.)
5. Any abnormal or immature leukocytes are noted and recorded.
6. The number of nucleated erythrocytes (if any) is noted and recorded. Red blood cell morphology is examined and abnormalities are noted and recorded.
7. Both the number and morphology of the platelets should be evaluated and recorded. Refer to Platelet Number and Morphology, which appears later in this chapter.

RED BLOOD CELL MORPHOLOGY

An examination of the morphology of the red blood cells is of utmost importance. In various anemias and other blood diseases, the red blood cells of the peripheral blood may display significant changes that will be of diagnostic importance to the clinician. The abnormal changes observed may be classified into four categories: differences in size, differences in shape, differences in intracellular content, and miscellaneous differences. The terms applied to each of the abnormalities will be defined and illustrated here and on subsequent pages.

Differences in Size (Anisocytosis)

When there is a *noticeable variation* in the size of the erythrocyte population on the blood smear, the term anisocytosis is used to describe this morphological occurrence. A moderate variation is normal, with the diameter of the cells ranging from 6.2 to 8.2 μ. Microcytes, macrocytes, and normocytes may be seen (Figure 14). Anisocytosis may be seen in many types of anemias and the thalassemias. In general, the more severe anemias are accompanied by the most severe anisocytosis.

1. *Normal Erythrocytes:* The normal red blood cell is called a *normocyte* or *discocyte*; therefore, a normal population of red blood cells seen on a blood smear are reported as being *normocytic*. Normal red blood cells range from 6.2 to 8.2μ in diameter. They are biconcave in shape and will appear round with a small central pale area. The discoid shape provides maximum surface area for the volume of the cell, thus gas exchange is easily facilitated across the membrane of the cell. The shape is not rigid, however, and the cell may assume different shapes when passing through small capillaries. There will be only slight variation in size (Figure 15).

2. *Microcytes:* Microcytes are erythrocytes that show a decrease in size. Red cells that have a diameter of less than 6.0 microns are termed *microcytic*. They are biconcave in shape, however, and have the central pale area. The MCV is usually below 75 fl in microcytosis. Microcytes are characteristically seen in iron-deficiency anemia and thalassemia.

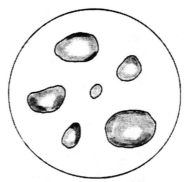

Figure 14. Anisocytosis. Redrawn from Barbara A. Brown: *Hematology, Principles and Procedures*, 2nd ed., 1976. Courtesy of Lea & Febiger, Philadelphia, Pennsylvania.

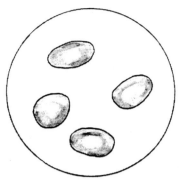

Figure 15. Normal erythrocytes. Redrawn from Barbara A. Brown: *Hematology, Principles and Procedures*, 2nd ed., 1976. Courtesy of Lea & Febiger, Philadelphia, Pennsylvania.

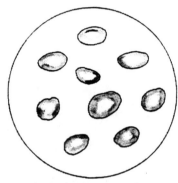

Figure 16. Microcytes. Redrawn from Barbara A. Brown: *Hematology, Principles and Procedures*, 2nd ed., 1976. Courtesy of Lea & Febiger, Philadelphia, Pennsylvania.

The cells may be hypochromic, as well as microcytic in these disorders. Microcytes that are not deficient in hemoglobin may be seen in some hemolytic anemias (Figure 16).

3. *Macrocytes:* Macrocytes are erythrocytes that show an increase in size. Red cells that have a diameter greater than 8.5 microns are termed *macrocytic.* They may be biconcave or spheroid in shape. Macrocytosis is seen normally in the newborn and infant, because reticulocytes are usually larger than adult red cells. Macrocytes may be seen when a large number of reticulocytes are present. The macrocytes will demonstrate polychromatophilia or diffuse basophilia. Macrocytosis is characteristic of vitamin B_{12} or folate deficiency. The MCV is usually above 105 fl (Figure 17).

Abnormalities in Shape (Poikilocytosis)

Poikilocytosis is the term used to indicate the presence of red cells of various shapes. Any number of morphological shape differences may be seen (Figure 18).

1. *Spherocytes:* Spherocytes are erythrocytes that have lost their bioconcave shape; they are spherical. They do not have the central pale area and appear more darkly stained (hyperchromic) on the blood smear. The *spherocyte* has a smaller surface area. Spherocytes may be

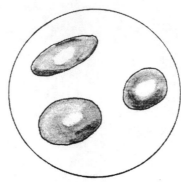

Figure 17. Macrocytes. Redrawn from Barbara A. Brown: *Hematology, Principles and Procedures*, 2nd ed., 1976. Courtesy of Lea & Febiger, Philadelphia, Pennsylvania.

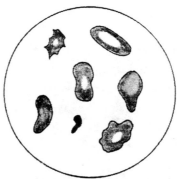

Figure 18. Poikilocytosis. Redrawn from Barbara A. Brown: *Hematology, Principles and Procedures*, 2nd ed., 1976. Courtesy of Lea & Febiger, Philadelphia, Pennsylvania.

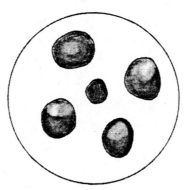

Figure 19. Spherocytes. Redrawn from Barbara A. Brown: *Hematology, Principles and Procedures*, 2nd ed., 1976. Courtesy of Lea & Febiger, Philadelphia, Pennsylvania.

microspherocytes (less than 6.0 microns) or macrospherocytes (greater than 8.5 microns). Prolonged storage of blood may result in the transformation of normocytes to spherocytes. Patients who have been transfused may show spherocytes on their blood smears. Spherocytes are characteristically seen in congenital spherocytosis, immune and mechanical hemolytic anemias, and in megaloblastic anemias as macrocytic spherocytes (Figure 19).

2. *Target cells (codocytes)*: Codocytes are erythrocytes that have a centrally

Figure A   Figure B

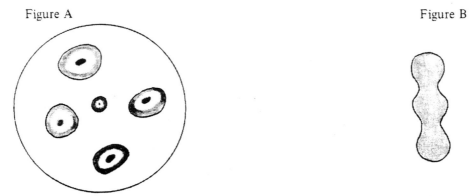

Figure 20. (A) Target cells. (B) Cross section of a target cell. Redrawn from Barbara A. Brown: *Hematology, Principles and Procedures*, 2nd ed., 1976. Courtesy of Lea & Febiger, Philadelphia, Pennsylvania.

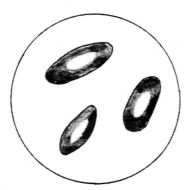

Figure 21. Elliptocytes. Redrawn from Barbara A. Brown: *Hematology, Principles and Procedures*, 2nd ed., 1976. Courtesy of Lea & Febiger, Philadelphia, Pennsylvania.

stained area, which is surrounded by a pale area that is, in turn, surrounded by a stained area. These cells actually resemble a target and result from insufficient hemoglobin content. *Codocytes* are common in hemoglobinopathies (Hbs, HbC, HbS-C, thalessemia, and sickle cell-thalassemia) (Figure 20).

3. *Elliptocytes (ovalocytes)*: Elliptocytes are erythrocytes that have an oval or elliptical shape. They are usually biconcave and, therefore, have the central pale area. True elliptocytosis is a congenital abnormality of red cells. The cause is unknown. Electron microscopy demonstrates bipolar aggregation of the hemoglobin. Acquired elliptocytosis may be present on blood smears in a variety of disorders (thalassemia, sickle cell trait, HbC trait, hemolytic anemia, etc.) (Figure 21).

4. *Burr Cells*: Burr cells have several pointed projections of the cell membrane. *Burr cells* occur when the cell membrane has been damaged by toxic substances or there are chemical changes in the plasma. Some hematologists prefer to use the term "schistocyte" instead of "burr cell." This deformity of the cell membrane occurs in many disorders, i.e. immune and mechanical hemolytic anemias, uremia, burns, kinase

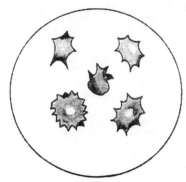

Figure 22. Burr cells. Redrawn from Barbara A. Brown: *Hematology, Principles and Procedures*, 2nd ed., 1976. Courtesy of Lea & Febiger, Philadelphia, Pennsylvania.

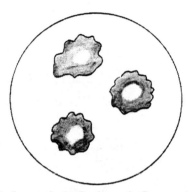

Figure 23. Crenated cells. Redrawn from Barbara A. Brown: *Hematology, Principles and Procedures*, 2nd ed., 1976. Courtesy of Lea & Febiger, Philadelphia, Pennsylvania.

deficiencies, bleeding peptic ulcer, aplastic anemia, and hypertension (Figure 22).

5. *Crenated cells*: Crenated cells have very irregular membrane projections. This is often due to improper technique in making the smear, faulty drying of the smear, or faulty Wright's stain. These errors result in the loss of intracellular water. The crenated cell projections appear rounded and short on the surface. No disorder is associated with the formation of *crenated cells*; they are regarded as insignificant (Figure 23).

6. *Schistocytes:* Schistocytes are fragmented erythrocytes that appear in a variety of conditions which cause tearing of the red cell membrane. *Schistocytes* may be an important indication of hemolytic anemia, whatever the cause: immune or mechanical. *Schistocytes* may also result from fibrin deposition in the microcirculation (as in DIC) or microangiopathic hemolytic anemia. *Schistocytes* are formed in patients with prosthetic heart valves, valvular stenosis, and hypertension. Patients with uremia, extensive burns, enzyme deficiencies, peptic ulcer, and aplastic anemia may also form schistocytes (Figure 24).

7. *Sickle cells (Drepanocytes)*: Drepanocytes are erythrocytes that have a sickled shape. Sickle cells are associated with Hemoglobin S disease but may be induced in some other hemoglobinopathies. Reducing agents

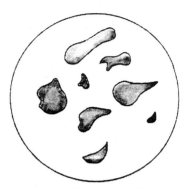

Figure 24. Schistocytes. Redrawn from Barbara A. Brown: *Hematology, Principles and Procedures*, 2nd ed., 1976. Courtesy of Lea & Febiger, Philadelphia, Pennsylvania.

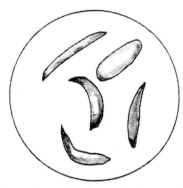

Figure 25. Sickle cells. Redrawn from Barbara A. Brown: *Hematology, Principles and Procedures*, 2nd ed., 1976. Courtesy of Lea & Febiger, Philadelphia, Pennsylvania.

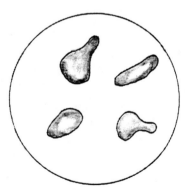

Figure 26. Tear drop cells. Redrawn from Barbara A. Brown: *Hematology, Principles and Procedures*, 2nd ed., 1976. Courtesy of Lea & Febiger, Philadelphia, Pennsylvania.

may cause sickling of erythrocytes due to reduction of the oxygen tension or pH. Sicklelike filaments, or holly-leaved projections are noted. They do not form rouleau; therefore, the sedimentation rate is usually low (Figure 25).

8. *Tear-drop cells (Dacrocytes)*: Dacryocytes are erythrocytes that are shaped like tear-drops. They are seen in several blood diseases and are quite commonly seen in pernicious anemia. The cause is unknown (Figure 26).

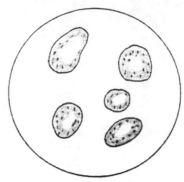

Figure 27. Basophilic stippling. Redrawn from Barbara A. Brown: *Hematology, Principles and Procedures*, 2nd ed., 1976. Courtesy of Lea & Febiger, Philadelphia, Pennsylvania.

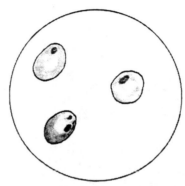

Figure 28. Howell-Jolly bodies. Redrawn from Barbara A. Brown: *Hematology, Principles and Procedures*, 2nd ed., 1976. Courtesy of Lea & Febiger, Philadelphia, Pennsylvania.

Abnormal Intracellular Inclusions

1. *Basophilic Stippling*: Basophilic Stippling is a condition in which the erythrocytes display several small blue-black granules. These granules are aggregates of heme precursors, iron, mitochondria, or ribosomes. They are seen in many diseases, but are of great diagnostic aid in identifying lead poisoning (Figure 27).

2. *Howell-Jolly Bodies*: Howell-Jolly Bodies are remaining fragments of the cell nucleus. They appear as round, darkly stained structures, usually singly in the cell. They are not refractile. This characteristic distinguishes them from superimposed granules (Figure 28).

3. *Siderotic Granules*: Siderotic granules are aggregates of iron that have not been utilized. The iron particles appear as blue-black dots on Wright's stained smears. Staining with Prussion blue stain is necessary for confirmation of iron. In Wright-stained cells, they appear faintly blue. The erythrocytes containing these iron structures are called siderocytes. A small number of normal adult erythrocytes and reticulocytes may demonstrate siderotic granules that probably represent iron in excess or not yet incorporated into hemoglobin. They are found in large numbers when there is ineffective hemoglobin synthesis and are absent when iron deficiency is present. (Refer to a color atlas for examples of siderotic granules.)

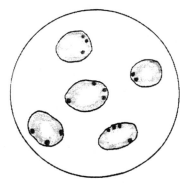

Figure 29. Heinz bodies. Redrawn from Barbara A. Brown: *Hematology, Principles and Procedures*, 2nd ed., 1976. Courtesy of Lea & Febiger, Philadelphia, Pennsylvania.

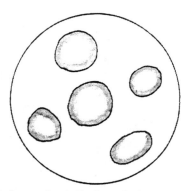

Figure 30. Hypochromia. Redrawn from Barbara A. Brown: *Hematology, Principles and Procedures*, 2nd ed., 1976. Courtesy of Lea & Febiger, Philadelphia, Pennsylvania.

4. *Heinz Bodies*: Heinz bodies are intracellular inclusions of denatured hemoglobin. They are single or multiple, refractile, irregular, or round bodies. They are not demonstrated by Wright's stain but are easily distinguished with crystal violet stain. The protein aggregates attach to the inner cell membrane, which renders the cell rigid and susceptible to lysis. They are produced by agents that are toxic to hemoglobin, as in many of the hemolytic anemias (Figure 29).

Miscellaneous Morphological Abnormalities

1. *Hypochromia*: This is a condition in which the erythrocytes have a very large area of central pallor due to decreased hemoglobin content. The greater the lack of hemoglobin, the more pale the cell will stain (Figure 30).
2. *Polychromasia*: Polychromasia is a condition in which the erythrocytes display varying degrees of pink-blue when stained. These calls are not yet fully mature and the remaining RNA causes the variation in color. (Refer to color atlas for examples of polychromasia.)
3. *Rouleau Formation*: Rouleau is the condition in which the erythrocytes are arranged in rolls or stacks. Rouleau results from imbalances in the concentration of plasma proteins or the presence of abnormal proteins. Erythrocytes are negatively charged and normally repel each

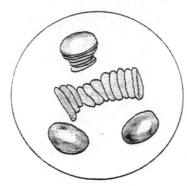

Figure 31. Rouleau. Redrawn from Barbara A. Brown: *Hematology, Principles and Procedures*, 2nd ed., 1976. Courtesy of Lea & Febiger, Philadelphia, Pennsylvania.

other. Proteins alter the zeta potential of cells, thus rouleau formation is increased (Figure 31).

4. *Superimposed Platelets*: Platelets that are lying on top of red cells should not be confused with red cell inclusions. Often the platelets will come to lie on top of an erythrocyte during the process of making the blood smear. To distinguish these, compare the platelet to those in surrounding microscopic fields. The superimposed platelet will generally have a unstained halo surrounding it. (Refer to a color atlas for examples of superimposed platelets.)

Discussion

1. When examining a blood smear, any of the preceding changes should be noted. However, an occasional abnormally shaped cell or a slightly large and/or slightly small cell may be seen normally and may be ignored. Crenated cells are not reported since they are artifacts.
2. Careful observation of several microscopic fields should be made prior to reporting the morphological findings.
3. Variations in size, shape, and staining quality may be graded as 1+, 2+, 3+, 4+; slight, moderate, marked; or other terminology common to the institution.

PLATELET NUMBER AND MORPHOLOGY

An examination of the morphology of the platelets is included as part of the blood smear examination. Platelet numbers are also examined; they are reported as increased or decreased. The following characteristics are examined:

1. *Size*: The normal platelet will vary from 1 to 4 microns in diameter. Larger platelets are thought to be more metabolically active, but large abnormal platelets are associated with a few rare diseases.
2. *Granules decreased or absent*: Platelet function is dependent upon substances located in the granules. Record the absence or decrease of platelet granules.
3. *Number per microscopic field*: Normally 10-25 platelets should be seen in a microscopic field containing 250-300 erythrocytes. Variation from

one field to another is largely due to the platelets' adherence to each other. They are often found in higher numbers near the end and edges of the smear. The number of platelets is estimated in each of 10 or more fields.

4. The number is recorded as normal, increased, or decreased and should be graded as slight, moderate, or marked.

STUDY QUESTIONS

1. Define:
   a. anisocytosis
   b. poikilocytosis
   c. polychromia
   d. hypochromia
   e. hyperchromia
2. List the four purposes of blood smear examination.
3. The size range for normal erythrocytes is _____.
4. Biconcave erythrocytes having a diameter of 6.0μ or less are called

   _____.

5. Biconcave erythrocytes having a diameter of 8.5μ or greater are called

   _____.

6. Define:
   a. spherocytes
   b. codocytes
   c. schistocytes
   d. drepanocytes
   e. siderocytes
7. Describe the following erythrocyte inclusions and indicate the composition of the inclusion structure:
   a. basophilic stippling
   b. Heinz bodies
   c. Howell-Jolly Bodies
   d. siderotic granules
8. Describe the following:
   a. burr cells
   b. crenated cells
   c. rouleau formation
9. Indicate a condition in which the following type of red cell abnormality might be found:
   a. schistocytes
   b. burr cells
   c. spherocytes
   d. macrocytes
   e. hypochromia
   f. rouleau formation
   g. elliptocytosis
10. Indicate the aspects of platelet morphology that are examined from the stained blood smear.

11. The pH of Wright's or Wright-Giemsa stain must be _____ for optimum staining.

12. Describe the properties of the Wright's or Wright-Giemsa stain that aid identification of the differential characteristics of cellular materials.

13. The substance used as a fixative in staining the blood smear is _____

14. In what position is the "spreader" slide placed before the smear is made?

15. The approximate angle between the spreader slide and blood smear slide is _____.

Chapter 5

DIFFERENTIAL CELL COUNTING

OBJECTIVES

The student will learn:

1. the procedure for differential cell counting.
2. the normal percentage values for leukocytes in peripheral blood.
3. the criteria that distinguish each type of leukocyte found normally in peripheral blood.
4. the constituents of Wright's or Wright-Giemsa stains that facilitate staining of blood cells.
5. the cytoplasmic substances in leukocytes that are distinguished by Wright's or Wright-Giemsa stains.
6. diseases in which the various leukocytes are found in increased or decreased numbers.
7. to calculate the absolute numbers of leukocytes.
8. the abnormal inclusions that appear in leukocytes.
9. the diseases that cause the development of abnormal leukocyte inclusions.

DIFFERENTIAL WHITE CELL COUNT

The diffential white cell (leukocyte) count is defined as the enumeration of the different types of white blood cells found in the blood. Since 100 white cells are counted in the process, the number of each type of cell is reported in percent. The report often plays a large role in the diagnosis of disease, as a particular cell type may show an increased percentage in a specific disease.

The differential is the last step in the examination of the blood smear. Erythrocyte morphology and platelet estimation and morphology are examined prior to performing the differential count.

There are six types of white blood cells that may *normally* be present in peripheral blood. These cells develop from immature precursors in the bone marrow and lymph nodes of the body. When mature or nearly mature, they enter the peripheral circulation. Leukopoiesis (formation of white blood cells) will not be discussed in this manual. For a detailed discussion of leukopoiesis, refer to any hematology textbook.

In identifying the various types of white cells, the following cellular aspects should always be kept in mind:

1. the size of the cell

2. the morphology of the nucleus
3. the morphology of the cytoplasm

A brief discussion of each of the six cell types will follow, with only the normal features of these cells being indicated.

MORPHOLOGICAL CHARACTERISTICS OF MATURE LEUKOCYTES

Granulocytes

There are three types of granulocytes that may be identified in the differential count: neutrophils, eosinophils, and basophils. Each cell is identified by the particular color of the specific (or secondary) granules located in the cytoplasm.

Neutrophils

The neutrophils are the most numerous of all the types of white cells. Approximately 55% to 70% of circulating leukocytes in adults are classified as neutrophils.

The characteristics of neutrophils follow:

1. The size is 10-15μ in diameter.
2. The cytoplasm is clear, is abundant, and does not usually take up any stain; rarely vacuoles may be seen.
3. The granules in the cytoplasm are small, numerous, fine, and take up a pink or lilac stain (neutral staining characteristics).
4. The nucleus is segmented, or lobated. Three to 5 segments or lobes are usually present, each segment being connected by a small filament. These cells are sometimes called polymorphonuclear (PMN) cells because of the various shapes of their nuclei.
5. The nucleus stains a deep purple-blue. The chromatin is densely clumped and a few small light areas (parachromatin) may be visible in the nucleus.
6. None to 5% of the neutrophils seen will be classified as *band neutrophils* because of the shape of the nucleus, which appears in a band form. The *band neutrophil* is less mature than the segmented form, but a few may normally be seen in peripheral blood. During the maturation process, the band nucleus gradually becomes segmented. The morphological characteristics of the band neutrophils are otherwise the same as the mature neutrophils, i.e. cytoplasmic characteristics, chromatin pattern, staining pattern. These band neutrophils are sometimes called "stab cells." The criterion for identification of bands has been a subject of much controversy. To be labelled a band there must be chromatin seen between two parallel sections of the nuclear membrane. In some laboratories, if a nucleus appears to be lobated but does not demonstrate a visible filament, the cell is classified as a segmented cell, the justification being that a filament must be present. Other hematologists do not agree with this assumption and believe that cells should be classified as segmented only when a *filament is visible*.
7. In rare instances neutorphils may appear with more than 5 segments. A congenital form of constitutional hypersegmentation has been

described in which most of the neutrophils have four lobes, with some having six or seven. This is a rare benign anomaly. In megaloblastic anemias hypersegmented neutrophils may be the first sign of the disease, even prior to any change in the MCV or other blood parameters.

Eosinophils

A second type of granulocytic white cell is the eosinophil, which means an attraction for eosin. In these cells, their basic contents attract the acid ions of the eosin stain. Thus, these cells display red to red-orange granules. Normally, 2-4% of the leukocyte population are eosinophils.

The characteristics of eosinophils follow:

1. Size range of 10-15 μ in diameter.
2. The cytoplasm is clear as in the neutrophilic series.
3. The granules in the cytoplasm are large red to red-orange granules that are uniformly distributed throughout the cytoplasm. They are often so numerous as to obliterate observation of nuclear morophology.
4. The nucleus (if observable) usually has only 2 lobes or segments that are separated by a thin filament. The chromatin is densely clumped and a few small parachromatin areas may be seen.
5. The nucleus stains a deep purple-blue color.
6. These cells are quite easily distinguished because of the large red to red-orange granules. One should not have difficulty differentiating them from neutrophils or basophils.

Basophils

The third type of granulocyte is the basophil, or the cell that attracts the basic dye of the stain. The acid contents of the granules in the cytoplasm attract the basic ions of the polychromed methylene blue of the stain. Thus, these cells display dark purple to purple-black granules. Normally 0-1% of the white cells are basophils.

The characteristics of basophils follow:

1. The size range is 10-15μ in diameter.
2. The cytoplasm is clear (if visible).
3. The granules in the cytoplasm are large, purple-blue to purple-black granules that are fairly uniformly distributed throughout the cytoplasm. The number of granules may be less than found in the eosinophils. They may, however, obliterate close observation of the nuclear morphology. These granules are water-soluble and may be washed out when stained.
4. The nucleus (if visible) may not be segmented but may be somewhat indented.
5. The nucleus stains a lighter purple-blue.
6. These cells are also quite easily distinguished from other cell types, thus, differentiation should not be difficult.

Lymphocytes

Lymphocytes are classified as mononuclear (one nucleus), non-granular cells. The mature lymphocyte may occur in any one of three sizes: small, medium, or large. The larger the lymphocyte, the more abundant the cytoplasm will be. Occasionally, the lymphocyte cytoplasm may contain a few small pink granules, often called "azurophilic" granules. In adults, the normal lymphocyte percentage will vary from 25% to 40%. Children and adolescents may have higher percentages of lymphocytes due to the fact that they are actively developing immunity to many organisms. Lymphocytes function in the immune process.

Characteristics of small lymphocytes follow:
1. The size variation is 8 to 10μ in diameter.
2. The amount of cytoplasm is very small, often only a thin ring around the nucleus or a small amount visible only on one side of the nucleus. Its color is medium blue.
3. The nuclear chromatin is very densely clumped. It stains dark purple-blue.
4. The nucleus is round or oval and may be slightly or deeply indented. It may be eccentric. No nucleolus is visible, due to the density of the chromatin. Parachromatin may be only vaguely visible or not at all. It stains deep purple-blue.

Characteristics of the medium-sized lymphocyte follow:
1. The size variation is from 8 to 14μ in diameter.
2. The more abundant cytoplasm stains pale to medium blue. A few pink granules may or may not be present in the cytoplasm.
3. The round or oval-shaped nucleus may be slightly or deeply indented and eccentric. It stains purple-blue. A nucleolus may be seen in larger cells. The nuclear chromatin is clumped but not as densely clumped as in the small lymphocyte.

Characteristics of the large lymphocytes follow:
1. The size ranges from 8 to 18μ in diameter.
2. An abundant amount of cytoplasm stains sky blue but may be medium blue. A few pink granules may or may not be present; their significance is unknown.
3. The nuclear shape is round or oval and may be slightly or deeply indented. It may be eccentrically located in the cell, and it stains purple-blue. The chromatin pattern of the nucleus is coarse and a few small lighter areas may be visible. A nucleolus may or may not be seen in larger cells.

Atypical Lymphocytes

Atypical lymphocytes are cells that are reacting to an abnormal stimulus. They probably should be referred to as "reactive lymphocytes" since they have accelerated RNA synthesis. They are seen in the blood in a variety of viral and nonviral conditions. They are popularly associated with infectious mononucleosis. The characteristics of atypical lymphocytes follow:
1. A large size, up to 20μ in diameter. Some may be smaller.
2. The cytoplasm is moderately to deeply basophilic, foamy, and occasionally contains vacuoles. The cytoplasm is abundant and stains more darkly near the cytoplasmic membrane.

3. The nuclear chromatin is usually less condensed and more homogeneous. A nucleolus may or may not be seen.

Monocytes

The monocytes are the largest of the peripheral blood cells. They are also classified as mononuclear and non-granulocytic, although there are many fine granules located in the cytoplasm. They arise from the same embryonic cell-colony as the granulocytic cells. These large phagocytic cells comprise approximately 4% to 8% of the white cell population.

The monocyte is easily identified if the blood smear is well prepared. If badly stained, the typcial features are lost and the characteristic fine granules may not be visible.

The characteristics of monocytes follow:

1. The size variation is 14 to 20 μ in diameter.
2. An abundant cytoplasm stains slate-grey to grey-blue. It is opaque. The presence of numerous very fine lilac granules gives a foamy, ground-glass-like appearance to the cytoplasm. There may or may not be vacuoles present in the cytoplasm.
3. The nuclear shape may be round, oval, kidney-shaped, folded, or slightly lobated. It is often folded over itself. It stains a blue to blue-purple. It is definitely lighter staining than in other cells. The chromatin pattern of the nucleus is usually loose, fine, and not clumped. It may appear to be arranged in fine strands. No nucleoli are usually visible; occasionally one may be seen.
4. The overall cell shape may be irregular due to the fact that the monocyte is very motile and phagocytic. The occasional presence of pseudopodia and/or vacuoles is evidence of these activities by the monocyte.

COUNTING THE WHITE BLOOD CELLS

Procedure

Once the different types of white blood cells have been identified and their characteristics learned, the cells must be counted to obtain the percentages of each cell type (differential white cell count).

1. Examine the blood smear under low power (10X objective).
   a. The red and white cells should be evenly distributed over the smear.
   b. If there are many white cells located near the peripheral edge of the smear in comparison to the number located nearer the center of the slide, distribution of cells is not good. This slide should be discarded and a new one made.
   c. Compare the number of white cells seen (in relation to the number of red cells) with the actual white cell count. The two should agree. If not, the white count should be repeated.
   d. Choose a portion of the smear where there is only a slight overlapping of the red blood cells (approximately 250-300 per field). Place a drop of immersion oil on the slide, after rotating the objective away from the slide. Now carefully change to the oil immersion objective (100X).

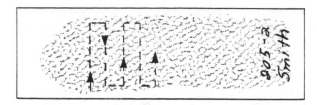

Figure 32. Movement of slide for differential cell counting.

2. Examine the red cell morphology, estimate the platelet numbers, examine the platelet morphology, and record these results.
3. Perform the differential cell count and examine the white cell morphology.
   a. Begin the counting in an area where the red cells are not too heavily overlapping. Gradually move the slide in the manner indicated in Figure 32, counting each white cell seen and recording each on a differential cell counter (or a piece of paper) until 100 cells have been counted.
   b. Any nucleated red blood cells seen should be recorded in a separate count and are not to be included as part of the differential count. It is very important that any nucleated red cells be reported, as these are not normally seen on peripheral blood smears. Newborn infants may show an occasional nucleated red cell, but they are considered abnormal findings on adult blood smears.
   c. While counting the white cells, make a note of any abnormalities present in the cells.

Discussion

1. Do not skip any cells; count all cells that are distinguishable. Occasionally a white cell may be ruptured during the process of making the smear. "Smudge" cells or "basket" cells result. These are not to be reported as part of the differential count. If high numbers are present, they should be reported as this may be indicative of increased cellular fragility.
2. Do not progress too far into the thick area of the slide when studying it. The morphological characteristics of the cells are too difficult to distinguish accurately in this area. Likewise, do not move too far into the thin edge of the smear because distortion of the cells, both red and white, will be present.
3. Report any abnormality of white cell morphology, such as toxic granulation, hypersegmented neutrophils, or heavily vacuolated cells.
4. When the white count is very low (below 1,000 per μl), it will be difficult to find 100 white cells on the blood smear. In this case, 50 white cells are differentiated and the results are multiplied by 2. A notation is made on the report that only 50 were counted.
5. The differential count is an indication of the percentage or relative number of each type of white cell. Occasionally, the physician may request an actual or absolute number of each white cell type. The absolute count is calculated as follows:

$$\begin{matrix} absolute\ number\ of \\ cells\ per\ \mu l \end{matrix} = \frac{\%\ of\ cell\ type\ in}{differential} \times white\ cell\ count$$

6. The following outline should be followed when studying the stained blood smear:
   a. Platelets
      (1) estimate number present
      (2) examine the morphology for abnormalities
   b. Red blood cells
      (1) examine the size
      (2) examine the shape
      (3) examine the hemoglobin content by observing the staining characteristics
      (4) examine the immaturity
      (5) examine for inclusion bodies
      (6) examine for the presence of rouleau formation
   c. White blood cells
      (1) estimate number present
      (2) perform the differential count
      (3) examine for morphological abnormalities
7. Do not hesitate to ask questions about the morphology or differentiation of cells that are questionable. The differential count is the most difficult of all the CBC procedures to master. No white cell is exactly like its sister cell, thus absolute characteristics do not exist. Much patience, practice, and persistence are necessary in learning to perform a good differential count.
8. Some diseases that show an increased number of a specified cell type are listed below.
   a. Segmented and band neutrophils are increased in:
      bacterial infections
      appendicitis
      granulocytic leukemia
   b. Eosinophils are increased in:
      asthma
      hay fever
      parasitic infections
      skin diseases
   c. Basophils are increased in:
      allergenic reactions
      granulocytic leukemia
   d. lymphocytes are increased in:
      viral diseases
      whooping cough
      infectious mononucleosis
      lymphocytic leukemia
   e. Monocytes are increased in:
      tuberculosis
      typhus fever
      brucellosis
      monocytic leukemia

9. The terminologies "shift to the left" and "shift to the right" are used to indicate changes from the normal percentages of the cell types. Shift to the left indicates the presence of immature forms of white cells, as seen in leukemias and infections. A shift to the right indicates the presence of hypersegmented neutrophils as might be seen in pernicious anemia.

10. The margin of error in a differential count ranges between $\pm 10\%$ and $\pm 15\%$.

MORPHOLOGICAL ABNORMALITIES OF LEUKOCYTES

Abnormalities of leukocyte morphology occur in a number of disorders or conditions. These result from abnormal maturation of the nucleus, cytoplasm, or both. A few of the abnormalities are discussed in this chapter. Refer to a color atlas for examples of abnormal conditions discussed below.

1. *Toxic granulation*: In severe infections and other toxic conditions, the neutrophilic bands and segmented cells may contain course, dark purple granules resembling the primary (non-specific) granules seen in more immature neutrophilic forms. In toxic conditions, the cytoplasm is altered so that a persistence of the primary lysosomes is seen. Toxic granulation is typically seen in hospitalized patients and is considered clinically insignificant. In healthy individuals it may be a sign of unsuspected infection or disease. It is important to distinguish acquired toxic granulation from abnormal granulation in severe congenital diseases such as Chediak-Higashi or storage disease syndromes. Toxic granulation disappears after the toxic condition ceases.

2. *Döhle Bodies*: In toxic conditions such as septicemia, burns, measles, or pneumonia, the cytoplasm of granulocytes may contain oval structures which are light blue or grey-blue in color. Döhle bodies are not abnormal inclusions but rather areas void or deficient of granules and rich in RNA. They may occasionally be seen in granulocytic leukemia, hemolytic anemia, and other myeloproliferative disorders. Döhle bodies disappear if the causative disorder is cured.

3. *May-Hegglin Anomaly*: Inclusions similar to Döhle bodies are seen in granulocytes, monocytes, and occasionally in lymphocytes in this congenital syndrome. The cytoplasmic inclusions persist throughout life, but the cells appear capable of normal function. Giant platelets, sometimes accompanied by thrombocytopenia, also characterize this disorder. Bleeding episodes, mild to severe, occur in one-third of the cases of May-Hegglin reported.

4. *Auer-Bodies*: Auer bodies are formed by coalescence of primary (nonspecific) granules within the endoplasmic reticulum. They appear rodlike, spindle shaped, oval, or round. On Wright's stained smears, they are red-purple in color. They are found only in granulocytic, monocytic, and myelomonocytic leukemia. True Auer bodies must give positive reactions to the cytochemicals characteristic of the inclusions found in acute granulocytic leukemia.

5. *Pelger-Hüet Anomaly*: The true Pelger-Hüet anomaly is a congenital anomaly characterized by decreased segmentation of the nuclei of

granulocytés, increased condensation of nuclear chromatic in all cells, and normal maturation of the cytoplasm. The anomaly is benign; the incidence is higher in Germany than in the U.S. The acquired pseudo-Pelger-Hüet has the same cellular characteristics. It is seen most often in chronic granulocytic leukemia but has been described in a variety of other disorders. The neutrophils have two lobes or none; the chromatin is very coarse, dense, and stains deeply. Cytoplasmic granulation is normal. *It is important that this anomaly be differentiated from a "shift to the left" seen in infectious diseases.*

6. *Giant Lysosomes*: The giant lysosomes present. in leukocytes in storage diseases and Chediak-Higashi syndrome are the result of enzymatic deficiencies that affect the metabolism of mucopolysaccharides or lipids. Accumulation of these substances in the cytoplasm form the large lysosomes characteristically seen in these diseases. Detailed discussion of these diseases is beyond the scope of this manual.

Discussion: Careful examination of the leukocytes for any of the previous abnormalities is necessary during observation of the blood smear. Any abnormality seen is reported along with the differential count.

STUDY QUESTIONS

1. Describe the procedure for differential cell counting.
2. Give the normal percentage values for the following cells:
   a. neutrophils _____
   b. lymphocytes _____
   c. monocytes _____
   d. eosinophils _____
   e. basophils _____
   f. neutrophilic bands _____
3. Describe the criteria that differentiate a band neutrophil from a segmented neutrophil.
4. The large granules of the eosinophil contain (acid, alkaline) substances that attract the (eosin, methylene blue) of the Wright's stain.
5. How many lobes of the nucleus does the mature neutrophil usually display?
6. The large granules of the basophil contain (acid, alkaline) substances, which attract the (eosin, methylene blue) of the Wright's stain.
7. Why do infants and preschool age children sometimes have a higher percentage of lymphocytes than neutrophils?
8. An increased percentage of _____ is usually associated with asthma, hay fever, and parasitic infections.
9. In appendicitis, one would expect to find an increased number of _____ and _____.
10. An increase in the number of white cells is called _____.
11. Calculate the absolute counts of the cells using the following values:
    WBC = 10,000 per μl
    neutrophils = 60%
    lymphocytes = 30%
    monocytes = 8%
    eosinophils = 2%

12. The lymphocyte has a:
    a. segmented nucleus
    b. kidney-shaped nucleus
    c. well-dispersed chromatin
    d. coarsely clumped chromatin
13. A few (1-5) small pink granules (sometimes called azurophilic granules) may be seen in the cytoplasm of the ＿＿＿＿＿＿＿.
14. Light grey or blue cytoplasm is characteristically seen in the ＿＿＿＿＿＿＿
15. What is meant by the expressions "shift to the left" or "shift to the right?"
16. Vaculoes may be seen in ＿＿＿＿＿＿ and ＿＿＿＿＿＿.
17. Toxic granulation may be seen in this type of white cell: ＿＿＿＿＿＿
18. A hypersegmented neutrophil has ＿＿＿＿＿＿ lobes and is most often associated with ＿＿＿＿＿＿.
19. An increased percentage of ＿＿＿＿＿＿ is usually associated with viral disease.
20. Describe the characteristics of an "atypical" lymphocyte.
21. List the content of the following abnormal leukocyte inclusions:
    a. toxic granulation ＿＿＿＿＿＿
    b. Döhle bodies ＿＿＿＿＿＿
    c. Auer bodies ＿＿＿＿＿＿
22. List a condition in which the following may be found:
    a. toxic granulation ＿＿＿＿＿＿
    b. Döhle bodies ＿＿＿＿＿＿
    c. Auer bodies ＿＿＿＿＿＿
    d. Pseudo Pelger-Hüet ＿＿＿＿＿＿
23. Döhle bodies and ＿＿＿＿＿＿ are found in May-Hegglin anomaly.
24. Giant lysosomes are seen in leukocytes in ＿＿＿＿＿＿ and ＿＿＿＿＿＿

Chapter 6

NONOPTICAL CELL COUNTING

OBJECTIVES

The student will learn:

1. the principle of nonoptical cell counting utilized in the operation of the Coulter-Counter.
2. the parts of the Coulter-Counter Model Fɴ.
3. the function of each of the parts of the Coulter-Counter Model Fɴ.
4. the procedure for operating the Coulter-Counter Model Fɴ.
5. the theory of "coincidence" and how this affects cell counting.
6. the proper dilutions used to count erythrocytes and leukocytes by the Coulter-Counter Model Fɴ.
7. to calculate the proper threshold dial setting for performing erythrocyte and leukocyte counts on the Coulter-Counter Model Fɴ.
8. the procedures for maintaining the quality of automated cell counting.
9. the cleaning techniques used to maintain the Coulter-Counter Model Fɴ.

AUTOMATION AND CELL COUNTING

Today's busy clinical laboratory is greatly indebted to Wallace and Joseph Coulter for the development and refinement of sophisticated methods for the counting of cells. Other industries requiring devices to enumerate particles of various kinds can also be grateful to the efforts of these two men.

Since 1956, several models of the Coulter Counter have been developed, from the original Model A to the very sophisticated current Model S Plus II, the latest model as of September 1981. Some model of Coulter Counter is the most frequently used instrument for cell counting in the clinical laboratory. There are other instruments currently available, but none so widely used as the Coulter-Counter. The Coulter Model F, Fɴ, and ZBI perform red and white cell counts and platelet counts. Additional attachments can be purchased that compute the hematocrit and MCV. The Model S gives all parameters of the count. The Model S is completely automatic from the time the undiluted blood sample is siphoned into the instrument until the results are printed out on a report form. When using the Model F, Fɴ, and ZBI, dilution of the blood samples and reporting of results are manual.

PRINCIPLE OF OPERATION OF THE COULTER COUNTER®

The Coulter Counter® (any model) is based on the principle that biological cells are poor electrical conductors, as compared with a saline solution. The Coulter uses a mercury-manometer-type syphon, which creates a vacuum in the system. The vacuum draws fluid through an orifice in a tube. If the fluid in a beaker is an electrolyte, an electrical current can be established between electrodes inside the tube and outside the tube. When the fluid (electrolyte) containing cells or particles is drawn through the orifice in the tube, the cells, being poor conductors of an electrical current, momentarily cause a decrease in the voltage. Each time a cell or particle passes into the path of the current, a voltage drop occurs. The magnitude, or size, of the voltage drop is proportional to the volumetric size of each cell. The voltage drops are fed into a complex electric circuit, which can discriminate between different amounts of voltage drops. The electric circuit then generates counting pulses for those cells larger than a certain size, or above a certain threshold level, thus counting the cells.

Summary

The principle involved in the operation of the Coulter instruments provides a nonoptical method for one-by-one sizing and counting of particles suspended in an electrolyte solution. As particles pass through an orifice within a specific path of current flow, displacement of an equal volume of electrolyte occurs, and the resistance in the path of the current changes. The magnitude of this change is proportional to the volumetric size of the particle. The number of changes in the current within a specific length of time is proportional to the number of particles within the solution.

THE MODEL Fɴ COULTER COUNTER

Only the parts and procedures for the operation of the Model Fɴ will be included in this section. Refer to Figures 33 and 35 for the parts discussed. Discussion begins at the top of the face of the instrument and concludes with the internal mechanisms.

Digital Readout Assembly

The digital readout consists of five glow tubes. The tube on the far right is the first to light up when counting begins. It represents the single particles, tube 2 represents the number of particles in tens, tube 3 in hundreds, tube 4 thousands, and tube 5 in ten-thousands. When counting stops, the numbers that are lit are read directly and the appropriate dilution correction made, if necessary. The instrument has been calibrated in such a way that the numbers indicated on the glow tubes are the number of cells (or particles) per μl, unless a different sample dilution has been used.

Monitoring System

The instrument has two monitors, the oscilloscope and the debris

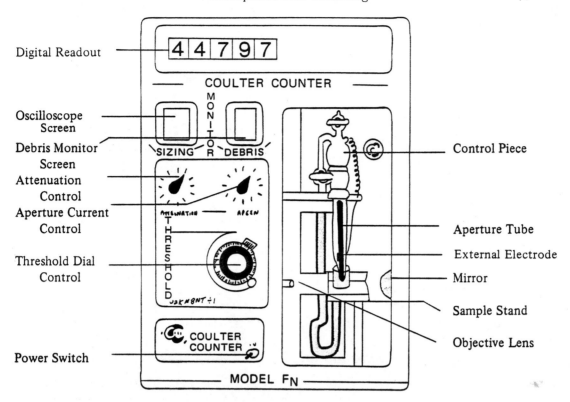

Figure 33. Coulter Counter®, Model FN, front view.

monitor. These provide the mechanism for the detection of irregularities during the count.

1. Debris monitor: This is an optical microprojection system, which gives a constant view of the tiny orifice (aperture) in the aperture tube, through which the sample solution passes. It consists of a projection lamp, mirror, and objective lens. The light from the projection lamp is reflected by the mirror onto the aperture. The objective lens focuses the aperture onto the debris monitor. This enables the operator to detect any debris that may block the aperture during a count. (If this occurs a small soft brush is used to brush away the debris.)

2. Oscilloscope: This screen gives an electronic measurement of each particle counted. Spikes, or pulses, are displayed on the screen each time a particle passing through the aperture causes a voltage drop. The height of each pulse is proportional to the volumetric size of the particle. This screen should be watched during the counting process to detect interfering debris or electrical interference, which will cause an abnormal pattern to be seen (Figure 34).

Sensitivity Controls

There are three sensitivity controls: the aperture current control, the attenuation control, and the threshold discriminator. The sensitivity control values are established through calibration of the instrument when it

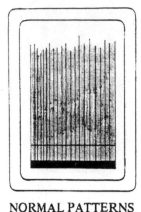 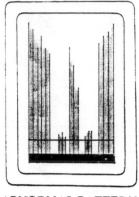

NORMAL PATTERNS   ABNORMAL PATTERNS

Figure 34. Oscilloscope patterns.

is first set up. Once established, these values are not changed as long as the electronics, manometer tube, and kind of particles being counted are not changed. Then recalibration is necessary. Periodic checks of the threshold discriminator should be done as a check on instrument operation.

1. *Aperture current control*: This controls the amount of current that passes between the two electrodes of the sample stand assembly. Increasing the current produces a larger voltage drop and higher pulse on the oscilloscope for a given size of cell. Decreasing the amount of current decreases the pulse height. Excessive current may damage biological cells, causing the cells to swell and produce larger voltage drops. Excessive current also decreases the ability of the instrument to measure smaller particles or cells.

2. *Attenuation control*: This control adjusts the overall sensitivity of the system, with regard to electronic amplification. It adjusts the electronic sensitivity of the Pre-Amp much as a volume control works on a radio.

3. *Threshold discriminator*: This control determines the lower size limit of the particle to be counted. Only voltage drops above the magnitude established as the lower limit will be recorded by the instrument.

Power Switch

The instrument should be turned on 10-15 minutes prior to use. The vacuum system must have time to build up.

Sample Stand Assembly

This assembly has several parts: the sample platform, aperture tube, two platinum electrodes, a control piece, and the mercury manometer.

1. *Sample platform*: This is a spring-activated platform on which the sample vial (or beaker) is placed. The aperture tube should be located close to the bottom of the vial, but not touching it.

2. *Aperture tube*: The aperture tube contains a small aperture (70 X

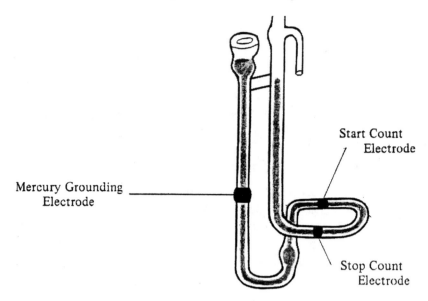

Figure 35. Mercury manometer with electrodes.

100 μ for red and white cells) through which the cells in the diluted sample pass. The debris monitor should be able to focus directly on the aperture. Controls for positioning the tube are located on the lower right side of the instrument.

3. *Platinum electrodes*: There are two electrodes: one inside the aperture tube (the internal electrode) and one outside the aperture tube (the external electrode). The external electrode must be immersed in the sample solution.

4. *Control piece*: This connects the aperture tube to the mercury manometer and contains two stopcocks: the flushing, or filling, stop-cock on the left and the vacuum control stopcock on the upper right. The filling (flushing) stopcock is used only when filling the aperture tube with fresh electrolyte, detergent solution, or other cleaning solutions. The vacuum control stopcock, when opened, creates a negative pressure, or vacuum, in the manometer, thus causing the mercury in the manometer to fall. The top of the control piece is connected to rubber tubing and a T tube, which is in turn connected to the vacuum regulator and to the waste flask. Behind the 2 stopcocks there is another opening that is connected to the electrolyte solution by a rubber tube.

5. *Mercury manometer*: This device controls the exact amount of diluted sample to be counted. For red and white counts a 500 lambda manometer is used. Thus, for those counts, exactly 0.5 ml of diluted sample is counted. There are three electrodes connected to the manometer. One electrode serves as a grounding contact. One electrode initiates the particle counting process and the third electrode stops the counting process as soon as 0.5 ml of diluted sample has been drawn through the orifice of the aperture tube (Figure 35).

Vacuum Pump

The vacuum pump regulates the mercury level in the manometer. The pump is controlled by the vacuum control regulator that is located above the pump. A piece of rubber tubing is attached to the vacuum pump. The vacuum limit of the pump is adjusted by this piece of tubing, which is pinched off at a predetermined length. This length should not be altered once it has been set.

Regulator Controls

There are three regulator controls located near the top of the right side of the instrument: the vacuum control regulator, which controls the vacuum pump; the light intensity control, which regulates the brightness of the projection lamp located behind the manometer; the dual volume control, which is positioned at the 100 or 500 lambda position depending upon the size of manometer being used. (For red and white cell counts, the control is placed in the 500 lambda position. For platelet counts a 100 lambda manometer is used and, therefore, the control is placed in the 100 lambda position.)

Aperture Positioning Controls

These two controls are located in the lower left area of the right side of the instrument. The entire sample stand assembly may be moved up and down, or forward and backward, for proper positioning of the aperture directly in front of debris monitoring system.

Vacuum Waste Flask

The vacuum waste flask is located on the right side of the instrument. It is connected to the vacuum pump and to the T tube of the control piece. The flask collects the waste solutions as they go through the instrument. *The waste level should always be kept below the overflow tube or it will be drawn into the vacuum pump.*

Oscilloscope Controls

The oscilloscope controls are located on the left side of the instrument. The intensity control regulates the brightness of the oscilloscope pulses. The horizontal position control centers the pulses on the screen. The vertical position control moves the pulses up or down on the screen.

Decade Sounder Device

The decade sounder system provides an auditory method of monitoring the counting process. Each time 1,000 particles are recorded by the instrument, a clicking noise is heard. The cadence of the clicks is uniform when the counting process is proceeding normally. If the aperture becomes clogged with debris, if there is electrical interference, or if there is some malfunction of the instrument, the cadence of the clicks will become irregular. The technologist will thus be alerted to the malfunction.

Operating Procedure

1. The instrument is turned on and allowed to warm up.
2. Using the Dade Dilutor, prepare two dilutions of the blood sample for the red and white cell counts.
   a. *White count dilution*: A 1:500 dilution is prepared as follows:
      (1) The knob on the top of the dilutor is turned to the 1:500 position.
      (2) The blood sample is mixed thoroughly.
      (3) Holding the sample under the probe of the dilutor, press the knob down and immediately release it.
      (4) The dilutor will now aspirate 20 microliters (0.02 ml) of the blood sample. Check the probe to make certain no air bubbles are present. Wipe the outside of the probe with a Kimwipe.
      (5) Place a clean accuvette under the probe.
      (6) Press the knob a second time and release it.
      (7) The dilutor will now dispense the blood with 10 ml of diluent (Isoton®, 0.85% sodium chloride, or other isotonic diluent). This gives the desired 1:500 dilution used for counting white cells.
      (8) Just prior to performing the count, add 3 drops of lysing agent to lyse the red cells and platelets in the dilution. (Zaponin®, Zap-Isoton®, or Zapoglobin®) Unless the red cells and platelets are destroyed, they will be counted along with the white cells.
      (9) When the dilution clears, the count may be performed.
   b. *Red cell dilution*: A 1:50,000 dilution is prepared as follows:
      (1) The red cell dilution is prepared from the white cell (1:500) dilution *prior to adding the lysing agent.*
      (2) The dilutor knob is turned to the 1:100 position.
      (3) The well-mixed 1:500 dilution is placed under the probe. Press the knob down and release it.
      (4) The dilutor will aspirate 100 microliters (0.1 ml) of the 1:500 dilution. Wipe the outside of the probe and make certain no air bubbles are present in the probe.
      (5) Place a clean accuvette under the probe. Press the knob down and release it.
      (6) The dilutor will dispense the 1:500 dilution with 10 ml of diluent into the accuvette. This results in the desired 1:50,000 dilution used for counting red cells.
      (7) Nothing is added to the 1:50,000 dilution. All cells (red, white, and platelets) will be counted when the red count is performed. However, the number of white cells and platelets are negligible in a 1:50,000 dilution.
3. Before the count is performed, check the background count of the isotonic diluent. This is to ensure that elevated counts are not due to contaminated diluent or vials. (Contamination of diluent or vials will increase the number of particles in the diluent, thus falsely increasing the counts.) The background count should be approximately 100 or less per μl to be good.
4. Mix the diluted sample well and place it on the sample stand, immersing the aperture tube and external electrode in the sample.

Move the vial so that the aperture tube touches the side of the beaker. This will facilitate a good projection of the aperture onto the debris monitor screen.

5. Open the vacuum control stopcock by turning it to a vertical position. When the stopcock is open, the external vacuum source initiates the flow of the diluted sample through the aperture and causes the mercury in the manometer to fall and assume a position in the open leg of the manometer slightly below the horizontal branch. A click will be heard when the mercury has fallen below the start contact electrode. At the sound of the click, the digital readout glow tubes will clear to 0. The baseline light on the oscilloscope screen will also appear with the sound of the click.

6. The stopcock is now closed to the horizontal position. The unbalanced mercury in the manometer will now start to assume its balanced position. As it rises, the siphoning of the diluted sample through the aperture continues. As the mercury in the open leg rises into the horizontal branch, it makes contact with a wire electrode, the start contact. This electrode energizes a high speed decade counter, which begins counting all pulses that reach or exceed the threshold level. A current runs through the aperture between the two electrodes of the aperture tube. When a cell (or particle) passes through the aperture, it causes a voltage drop (because it is a poor electrical conductor), which is then registered on the digital readout tubes. The siphoning and counting continues until, a few seconds later, the mercury column makes contact with a second wire electrode, the stop contact, which stops the counter. The siphoning action continues until the mercury column comes to rest at a level near that of the mercury in the reservoir— that is, the balanced position. The grounding electrode in the manometer provides a ground return path for the start and stop electrodes.

7. Observe the oscilloscope and debris monitor screens for irregularities during the count. If debris clogs the aperture, lower the sample stand and gently brush the aperture with a small camel hair brush to remove the debris. Raise the sample stand, immersing the aperture tube and external electrode, and start the count again from step 5.

8. Record the count shown on the digital readout, reading from left to right. Round off the count to the nearest hundred. Perform two additional counts on the same sample. These counts should agree within 200-300 cells. Average the three counts to obtain the count. The count as it appears on the digital readout represents the number of white cells per μl in the blood sample. The instrument is calibrated to give the direct count using a 1:500 dilution. The red cell count readout must be multiplied by 100 to obtain the number of red cells per μl in the blood sample. (A 1:100 dilution was made when the red count was set up.)

9. Coincidence correction is now made, if needed, using the coincidence chart obtained with the Coulter-Counter. This correction is necessary because two or more cells may pass through the aperture simultaneously, producing only one current change and, thus, only one count. The manufacturer has mathematically computed the number of times two

or more cells pass through the aperture in a specific count and, using the data, has prepared a chart to use for count correction. The coincidence is negligible in counts below 10,000 per μl and, therefore, correction is not necessary.

Discussion

1. When changing from white cell to red cell samples, flush the aperture tube with diluent before counting the red cells. A carry-over of lysing agent from the white cell sample will lyse some of the red cells in the red cell sample and, thus, reduce the count.

2. When the electric current between the aperture tube electrodes changes due to a nonconducting cell or particle passing through it, the changing electrode signal is amplified and connected to the threshold discriminator. The threshold discriminator is set to give an output pulse only if the amplified electrode signal rises above a preset value. The purpose of the threshold discriminator is to reject signals from the electrodes that are below those expected from the particles being counted; therefore, particles smaller than the particles one wants to count are not counted. The pulses from the threshold discriminator are amplified and passed through the count control circuits to the digital readout assembly. The count control circuits allow pulses to pass to the digital readout assembly only while the prescribed volume of electrolyte is being passed through the aperture. The volume of electrolyte passed through the aperture is controlled by the manometer. As the unbalanced mercury initiates the siphoning and contacts the start count electrode, an electric circuit is completed, which causes the count control circuits to allow pulses to pass to the decade counter assembly and be counted. When the mercury column has moved the distance required to have siphoned the prescribed electrolyte volume through the aperture, a second electric circuit is completed (as the mercury contacts the stop electrode) that causes the count control circuits to stop pulses from passing to the decade counter. The aperture tube electrode signals fed to the threshold discriminator are also amplified and presented on the oscilloscope screen. The oscilloscope shows the changing electrode signals as particles pass through the aperture. The pulses seen are those of all signal amplitudes, those greater than the threshold level and those less than the threshold level.

3. Always make sure the external electrode is fully immersed in the sample vial. In addition, make sure the electrode is not blocking the objective lens so that the aperture can be seen on the debris monitor.

4. To avoid interference during the counting procedure, keep your hands away from the instrument. Moving or jarring the instrument or the sample vial will cause erratic oscilloscope patterns and inaccurate test results. In case of electrical interference, check the grounding mechanism or operation of other electrical equipment in the room. It may be necessary to install a completely separate electrical circuit for the counter if electrical interference from outside sources persists.

5. It is not necessary to have a different threshold dial setting for red and white cell counts. Once the dial setting has been established, it may

be left in that position unless the electronics or the manometer are changed.

6. Extremely high or low counts should be repeated at different dilutions to give greater accuracy. For high counts (above 75,000) increase the amount of diluent used. For low counts, increase the volume of blood used in the dilution. Dilution corrections must then be made accordingly.

7. When the Counter is not in use, it should be left with either Isoterge® (a detergent cleaning solution) or electrolyte solution in it. If the instrument is not used daily, Isoterge® should be left in it. Occasional cleaning (to remove protein build-up in the aperture tube assembly) is best done by using a weak (5%) bleach solution. This is flushed through the instrument in the same manner as Isoterge® or electrolyte solution. If Isoterge® or bleach solution is used, the aperture tube must then be rinsed thoroughly with the electrolyte (diluent) prior to counting.

8. The counting cycle (from start contact electrode to stop contact electrode) should be approximately 12 to 15 seconds for accurate results. Less than 12 seconds may indicate a broken aperture. A cycle greater than 15 seconds usually indicates a blocked or dirty aperture or a dirty manometer and mercury.

9. A very important part of the quality control of the Coulter is regular cleaning maintenance. With periodic cleaning of the aperture tube and the manometer, the instrument will operate accurately and effectively. The vacuum pump should be oiled periodically with non-detergent #20 engine oil to keep it operating efficiently. Refer to the Operator's Manual for instruction in assembly and maintenance of the Coulter Counter. Problems are minimal with the Model Fɴ. When they do occur, the Coulter repairman should be notified.

Reference Controls

Commercially prepared Reference Controls or Reference cells for hematology are available from a number of reputable companies. Coulter Diagnostics manufactures reference cells called 4C. These cells may be purchased with normal CBC parameters and with abnormal CBC parameters. The 4C shelf-life is 30 days and may be used for quality control purposes during this time unless deterioration occurs. Dade's reference cells are called CH-60, and have a shelf-life of 60 days. Normal and abnormal CH-60 cells may be purchased for quality control usage. Pfizer standards, Celltrol and Leukotrol, are also available.

Normal and abnormal reference controls must be run daily and the values plotted on a quality control log or assay sheet. Trends and shifts resulting from instrument or technologist malfunction or error, reagent contamination, or reference cell deterioration can thus be observed and the cause determined and corrected before patient tests are performed.

Additional Quality Control Measures

1. The stained blood smear examination should agree with the instrument count.

a. Low red cell counts may be the result of rouleau formation, which will be obvious during the smear examination. In blood samples having rouleau formation, the aggregates of red cells will pass through the aperture and be recorded as one cell, thus lowering the count. In case of rouleau, an exact aliquot of the blood sample is centrifuged and the plasma removed. The cells are then washed at least three times to remove any remaining plasma, and the volume of the original aliquot restored by adding 0.85% sodium chloride. The red cells/sodium chloride mixture is then thoroughly mixed and the count performed on this sample as usual. (Removal of the plasma proteins prevents rouleau formation.)

b. The instrument white count can also be checked by examining the stained blood smear. High and low instrument counts should correspond with the numbers observed on the smear.

2. On a weekly basis several blood samples should be saved and refrigerated overnight. The next morning, these samples should be warmed to room temperature and the red and white cell counts repeated. These counts should not change appreciably from the counts of the previous day if quality control has been maintained.

3. On a weekly basis several normal freshly drawn blood samples should be counted to assure quality control. If the instrument, reagents, technologist, etc., yield reliable counts on normal blood samples, the accuracy of the results is dependable.

ADDITIONAL AUTOMATED CELL COUNTERS

There are several automated instruments that also operate on the electrical conductivity principle: Royco Instruments Division, Clay Adams (Division of Becton, Dickinson and Co.), and Hycel, Inc., have all developed instruments that employ the electrical conductivity principle for cell counting. Fisher Scientific Company, Ortho Diagnostics Instruments, Technicon Instruments Corporation, and others have developed instruments that optically count cells by occluding or reflecting a beam of light, by dark field illumination, or by light scattering principles. These instruments will not be discussed in detail. Information regarding these systems can be obtained from the manufacturers.

CALIBRATION OF THE COULTER COUNTER® MODEL F$_N$, F, ZBI

Calibration of the Coulter Counter Model F$_N$ is done when the instrument is first installed in the laboratory. The formula for determining the calibration constant of the instrument follows:

$$K = \frac{V}{A \times B \times T_L}$$

where K = the calibration constant
A = aperture current
B = attenuation switch setting
T$_L$ = threshold setting for half counts
V = average volume of the known system

Once the calibration constant has been determined, it remains the same unless the aperture tube, manometer, or any of the electronics are changed. When this occurs, K must be recomputed.

Knowing the calibration constant one can determine the average volume of an unknown system (average volume of an unknown red cell blood sample) by changing the above formula to read:

$$V = KABT_L$$

The last step in the calibration process is to establish the threshold control setting to be used for counting the desired particle. For routine cell counting, the threshold control is left at a sufficiently low setting to count the smallest cells likely to be encountered and need not be reset for different samples. A periodic check of the control setting, using the reference cells, provides an additional measure for quality control.

Establishing the Threshold Control Setting

In establishing the threshold control setting, the value of each division of the control dial (threshold factor) must first be determined. Use of a standard of known measurement is necessary in this process. The reference cells (4C, CH-60, etc.) provide the system of known measurement, which is employed to determine the value of each of the small divisions of the control dial. Once this value has been established, the control setting for the lower size limit of the cells to be counted can be determined. The proper threshold control will eliminate unwanted counting of particles less than the size of the red cells and white cells (debris and electrical interferences) but will allow counting the smallest red and white cells.

The formula for computing the threshold factor (value of each division of the threshold dial) follows:

$$T_F = \frac{V}{T_L}$$

> *where T_F = threshold factor*
> *V = average volume of known system (MCV of reference cells)*
> *T_L = threshold setting for half counts*

Equipment and Reagents

1. Isoton® or other isotonic diluent (electrolyte)
2. dirt free vials
3. dilutor or appropriate pipets to make dilutions
4. reference cells
5. applicator sticks
6. Kimwipes
7. Coulter Counter Model, F, F_N, ZBI

Principle

A very weak suspension of the reference cells is prepared and the number of cells in the suspension is determined at three low control settings. The counts are averaged and the control setting is increased until only one-half of the cells are counted by the instrument. This is the half-count and represents the larger one-half of the cells in the suspension. The smaller cells have not been counted because their sizes did not reach the limit established by the threshold control when it was increased upward. The threshold control setting for the half count represents the MCV of the cells in the suspension (one-half of the cells are smaller than this volume and one-half of the cells are larger than this volume). The reference volume is known, the threshold setting for the half count has been established, and the threshold factor (T_F) can then be determined using the formula.

Procedure

1. Thoroughly mix the vial of reference cells, which have a known MCV.
2. Prepare a dilute sample (approximately 20,000 cells) of the reference cells in electrolyte. This can be accomplished by lightly touching a bubble in the reference cell vial with an applicator stick, submersing it in the electrolyte solution, and swishing it in the solution to remove the cells from the stick.
3. Turn the threshold control dial to a setting of 5 to check the number of cells in the prepared sample. If too many cells (above 23,000) or too few cells (below 18,000) are present, adjust the sample accordingly. Record the count.
4. Take two additional counts of the sample, at dial settings of 8 and 1. Record these counts.
5. Add the three counts and average them. This is the *average original count*.
6. Divide the average original count by 2 to obtain the half count.
7. Rotating the threshold dial upward, obtain the threshold setting at which the half count was reached.
8. Using the formula, compute the value of each of the divisions of the threshold dial control (threshold factor).

Example:

threshold dial setting 5 = 20,000 cells
threshold dial setting 8 = 19,500 cells
threshold dial setting 1 = 21,000 cells
          Total   = 60,500 cells

$$average\ original\ count = \frac{60.5}{3} = 20.2\ (nearest\ tenth)$$

$$half\ count = \frac{20.2}{2} = 10.1$$

threshold setting at which 10,100 cells were counted = 40
MCV of known system (reference cells) = 80 fl

$$T_F = \frac{MCV}{T_L}$$

$$T_F = \frac{80}{40}$$

$$T_F = 2\mu$$

Thus each increment of the threshold dial has a value of $2\,\mu$. Each time the dial is increased upward by 1 division, the diameter of the particle, which will be counted by the instrument, is increased by 2 microns.

9. The threshold dial setting for counting red and white blood cells is determined by dividing the threshold factor into the average original count.

Example:
threshold factor $= 2\mu$
average original count $= 20.2 \times 10^3$
threshold setting
for counting red $= \dfrac{20.2}{2} = 10.1$ *or 10*
and white cells

Discussion

1. The reference cells must be brought to room temperature prior to preparing the dilute suspension.
2. At the three different dial settings (5, 8, 1), there is not a great variation in the number of cells being counted by the instrument. Thus, the threshold setting could be varied considerably without affecting the count.
3. A large amount of dilute suspension should be prepared so that sufficient sample is available for all the counts.

STUDY QUESTIONS

1. What is the principle involved in particle counting by the Coulter Counter®?
2. A solution capable of conducting an electrical current is called _____.
3. What is the function of the threshold control?
4. What is the purpose of having the external and internal electrodes attached to the aperture tube?
5. The size of the orifice in the aperture tube used to count red and white cells is _____.
6. The amount of current flowing between the two aperture tube electrodes is controlled by the _____. The optimum setting is _____.
7. What is the function of the manometer?
8. The counting process is initiated by _____.
9. The particle suspension is drawn through the aperture by _____.
10. What is the theory of coincidence in particle counting?
11. What is the function of the oscilloscope?
12. Indicate the events that follow the opening of the vacuum control stopcock.
13. True or false: The height of the pulses on the oscilloscope screen are directly proportional to the volumetric size of the particles being counted.
14. The usual dilutions for counting red and white cells in the Model Fɴ are:
a. red cell dilution _____.

b. white cell dilution _____.

15. Give the volumes of blood and diluent required to prepare the previous dilutions:

    a. red cell dilution_____ blood _____ diluent

    b. white cell dilution _____ blood _____ diluent

16. What volume of particle suspension is counted by the Coulter Counter® during each counting cycle?

17. Write the formula for determining the following:

    a. calibration constant

    b. threshold factor

    c. MCV of blood sample (knowing T_F)

18. List four ways of monitoring the quality of particle counting.

19. In event that the white count is above 73,000 per μl, what adjustment is needed to give a more accurate count?

20. The manometer size used in counting red and white cells is _____.

21. What is the purpose of the objective lens that is focused on the aperture?

22. Why is "coincidence correction" made?

Chapter 7

MISCELLANEOUS TESTS

OBJECTIVES

The student will learn:

1. the normal values for the sedimentation rate for the following:

   Wintrob Method   *Westergren Method*

   Men   Men

   Women   Women

   Children   Children

2. the factors and/or diseases that affect the sedimentation rate of erythrocytes.

3. the definition of viscosity and density.

4. the three purposes for determining the sedimentation rate of erythrocytes.

5. the three stages in the sedimentation rate of erythrocytes.

6. the properties of new methylene blue stain.

7. the cytochemical properties of reticulocytes.

8. the importance of performing a reticulocyte count.

9. pathological conditions in which increased or decreased reticulocyte counts may be found.

10. the procedure for performing the reticulocyte count.

11. the normal values for a reticulocyte count.

12. the normal values for a platelet count.

13. three methods for performing platelet counts.

14. pathological conditions in which increased or decreased platelet counts may be found.

15. how the reliability of the platelet counts may be checked.

16. the indirect method (Fonio) of platelet counting.

SEDIMENTATION RATE (ESR)

If blood is drawn and mixed with an anticoagulant so that it remains fluid, the erythrocytes will gradually settle to the bottom of the container. In most normal persons sedimentation takes place slowly, but in a variety of disease states the rate is rapid and in some cases, proportional to the severity of the disease. Measurement of the sedimentation rate has become a helpful laboratory test in diagnosing occult disease or confirming and following the course of manifest disease. The sedimentation rate is expressed as the distance (in millimeters) that erythrocytes fall per unit of time (usually 1 hour).

The ESR is essentially a rough measure of abnormal concentration of fibrinogen and serum globulins. It measures the suspension stability of erythrocytes.

It has been found that erythrocytes settle more rapidly in the blood of women than of men and much more rapidly after the third or fourth month of pregnancy. Normal rates return after one month post partum. Increased rates are also observed in tuberculosis and other chronic infectious diseases, in which it increases with the activity of the disease; in cancer; in various connective tissue diseases, such as rheumatic fever and rheumatoid arthritis; in localized acute inflammation in which the rate appears to increase with the leukocyte count; and in dysproteinemias, such as multiple myeloma.

The viscosity, density, and mass of a substance have varying effects upon the velocity (a time rate of change of position) of the particles in that substance. The sedimentation velocity (rate) of erythrocytes in blood is affected by these factors as well. The discussion that follows demonstrates the direct and inverse relationships to viscosity, density, and mass as they affect the sedimentation of red cells. Each theoretical relationship is explained.

Plasma Factors

An increase in the ESR is favored by elevated plasma proteins, especially fibrinogen and somewhat less by elevated globulins.

In normal blood, erythrocytes suspended in plasma form few aggregates. The mass of the sedimenting particle is small, and the sedimentation rate tends to be low. In abnormal blood, rouleau formation or erythrocyte aggregation may take place, increasing the particle mass and the sedimentation rate. Rouleau formation depends largely upon the protein composition of the plasma, particularly with regard to fibrinogen and globulins. Erythrocytes are negatively charged and normally repel each other. Abnormalities of plasma composition alter the electrical charges. As a result, the disc-shaped erythrocytes stack into rouleau or form aggregates. In either case, there will be an increase in sedimentation rate due to a larger particle size and weight.

Number of Erythrocytes

The sedimentation rate is inversely proportional to the density of the blood. Density is defined as the number of particles per unit of volume. When the number of erythrocytes per unit volume of blood is greater or less than normal, the sedimentation rate is modified. In severe anemia the ESR is very rapid, due to the greater ease of settling of a small number of particles in a large volume of fluid. The blood sample is less viscous (less friction between cells as they slide past each other). The converse is true in polycythemia. The increased crowding of the settling particles tends to retard their fall due to the increased friction created by the crowded cells.

Size and Shape of Erythrocytes

Macrocytes fall more rapidly and microcytes less rapidly than normal erythrocytes. The larger the cells, the smaller the surface in relation to the volume. The sedimentation rate is directly proportional to the weight of the cell and inversely proportional to the surface area. When rouleau formation occurs, the aggregate of erythrocytes has increased weight but decreased surface area. This results in acceleration of the ESR. Abnormally shaped red cells, which do not form rouleau, will cause the ESR to be slowed down. Sickled cells and spherocytes are examples.

Position of the Tube

In all methods, it is extremely important to keep the tube exactly perpendicular. Small degrees of tilting have a marked accelerating effect on the ESR. This is due to the settling of cells to one side of the tube, affording the plasma easier displacement upward. Special racks are used to keep tubes vertical.

Anticoagulant Used

Anticoagulants may affect the size of the erythrocyte and thus alter the sedimentation rate. Dry potassium or sodium oxalate may shrink red cells as much as 10 percent. Heparin causes minimum shrinkage. Liquid sodium citrate and EDTA have the least effect on cell size. When considering the convenience of being able to use EDTA—anticoagulated blood for cell counting and hematocrit determinations, as well as for determining the sedimentation rate, it would seem expedient to draw the samples in EDTA. However, in 1973 the International Committee for Standardization in Hematology established a "standard" method using the Westergren tube but specified that blood samples be drawn into liquid sodium citrate anticoagulant. This blood is only useful for the sedimentation rate determination. Some hematologists still prefer the EDTA samples for convenience. Blood samples drawn in EDTA may be diluted with sodium citrate or sodium chloride and then the sedimentation rate can be determined. Results are reproducible and are almost identical with those obtained by the standard Westergren method.

Effects of Temperature

Minor fluctuations in room temperature do not greatly affect the ESR. It has been shown that if blood is at refrigerator temperature, the ESR is significantly decreased, probably because of the increase of plasma viscosity. It is important, therefore, to have the blood at room temperature before performing the test.

Effect of Delay in Performing Test

The ESR remains unchanged for 12 hours after the blood has been drawn, if the blood has been drawn in potassium EDTA. If the blood is drawn in double oxalate, there is a significant reduction in the ESR after 3 hours.

Effect of Changes in Plasma Composition

The plasma composition is by far the most important factor affecting the ESR. The plasma proteins and colloids affect the degree of rouleau and aggregate formation and, therefore, the sedimentation rate. As a result of studies, the important proteins are fibrinogen, alpha-2 globulin, and alpha-1 globulin; an increase in these proteins produces an increased ESR. Of the three, fibrinogen is the most important. The ESR cannot, however, be used to estimate increases or decreases in any given fraction. It is significant, however, that the sedimentation rate is increased in those diseases in which changes in the protein pattern can be expected.

Clinical Correlation

Women show a higher ESR than men; children have a lower rate than adults. In pregnancy, the ESR begins to increase at about the third month and remains elevated until about 3 weeks after delivery. This is due to a greater increase in plasma volume than in erythrocyte mass. As an aid to *differential diagnosis*, the ESR is very useful. An accelerated rate suggests organic disease rather than a functional disorder, an inflammatory condition rather than a tumor, and malignancy rather than a benign tumor. The ESR is elevated in myocardial infarction but normal in angina pectoris; it is elevated in rheumatic fever, rheumatoid arthritis, tuberculosis, gouty or gonococcal arthritis but not in osteoarthritis; it is generally normal in cirrhosis of the liver but may be elevated in carcinoma of the liver. The ESR has proved its chief usefulness as a guide to the *progress of an infection and marking a point of change.*

Normal values for the sedimentation rate are listed below:

	Wintrobe	*Westergren*
men:	0-9 mm/hr	0-15 mm/hr
women:	0-15 mm/hr	0-20 mm/hr
children:	0-13 mm/hr	0-10 mm/hr

Modified Westergren Method

Equipment and Reagents

1. sodium chloride, 0.85% or 3.8% sodium citrate
2. Westergren pipet, which is calibrated from 0 to 200 mm and holds 1.0 ml of blood
3. Westergren rack
4. plain 13 × 100 test tubes

Principle

The blood is collected in EDTA anticoagulant. Since undiluted blood is too viscous for this test, the well-mixed blood is diluted with 0.85% sodium chloride or sodium citrate. The Westergren pipet is filled, and the pipet is allowed to stand for exactly one hour. The number of millimeters the red cells have fallen during the one hour period is the sedimentation rate.

Procedure

1. Place 0.5 ml of 0.85% sodium chloride in a test tube (or 0.5 ml of 3.8% sodium citrate).
2. Add 2.0 ml of well-mixed whole blood to the test tube containing the sodium chloride. (The blood sample should be at room temperature.)
3. Mix the contents of the tube for 2 minutes.
4. Fill the Westergren pipet to exactly the 0 mark, making certain no air bubbles are present in the column. (The blood may be drawn above the 0 mark, the outside of the pipet may be wiped, and the blood may then be allowed to drain out to the 0 mark.
5. Place the pipet evenly in the grooves of the Westergren rack. (A piece of Parafilm® may be placed over the groove of the rack to facilitate easier cleaning of the rack following the test.)
6. Allow the pipet to stand for exactly 1 hour.
7. At the end of the 1 hour, record the number of millimeters that the red cells have fallen. This reading is the ESR in millimeters per hour.

Landau-Adams Method

The Landau-Adams method may be used to determine the ESR when only capillary blood samples are available.

Equipment and Reagents

1. sterile lancets, alcohol swabs, sterile gauze, and other equipment necessary for capillary punctures
2. Landau microsedimentation pipets, with suction attachments
3. 5% sodium citrate
4. Landau sedimentation rack

Principle

The same principle applies in this method as in the Modified Westergren Method.

Procedure

1. Draw 5% sodium citrate solution up to the first line of the microsedimentation pipet.
2. From a capillary puncture, draw blood into the pipet until the fluid reaches the upper mark.
3. Wipe the end of the pipet. Draw the blood into the bulb, leaving a few millimeters in the stem to avoid air bubbles.
4. Mix the contents of the pipet. Slowly transfer the blood back into the stem, then draw the blood back into the bulb and mix again. Repeat, mixing three times in all, ending with the blood in the stem. The blood column may be at any point in the stem, but must not be in the tip. No bubbles should be in the column.
5. Place a finger over the tip of the pipet, remove the suction device, and place the pipet in the special sedimentation rack for 60 minutes.
6. Read at end of 60 minutes.

Wintrobe and Landsberg Method

This method is not recommended as an acceptable measure of the sedimentation rate or erythrocytes.

Equipment and Reagents

1. Wintrobe tube, which is calibrated from 0-100 mm, and holds 1.0 ml of blood
2. Wintrobe tube rack
3. Wintrobe pipets for filling the Wintrobe tubes

Principle

The blood is collected in EDTA anticoagulant. The well-mixed whole blood is placed in a Wintrobe tube and allowed to stand for exactly 60 minutes. The number of millimeters the red cells have fallen during this period of time is the ESR.

Procedure

1. With the Wintrobe pipet, fill a Wintrobe tube to exactly the 0 mark with the well-mixed whole blood. (The blood should be at room temperature.)
2. Place the tube upright in the leveled Wintrobe rack.
3. Allow the tube to stand for exactly 1 hour.
4. At the end of the hour, record the number of millimeters that the red cells have fallen. This result is the ESR in millimeters per hour.

Discussion

1. The International Committee for Standardization in Hematology has recommended the Westergren Method as the basic for an acceptable standard method. The Modified Westergren is more convenient since it allows the ESR to be performed from the same tube of blood as is used for other hematologic studies.
2. There are three stages in the sedimentation rate of red blood cells:
   a. *Initial phase* of aggregation: During this period there is rouleau formation and the sedimentation rate is slow; it lasts about 10 minutes.
   b. *Rapid settling phase*: Rouleau formation is maximized and sedimentation occurs at a constant rate; it lasts about 40 minutes.
   c. *Packing phase*: Third and last phase, which continues for the remainder of the hour and continues thereafter for a period of time.
3. It was formerly the custom to make a correction of the sedimentation rate for anemia. It is now generally agreed that there is little merit in reporting corrected sedimentation rates. The ESR is interpreted according to its relationship to the anemia.

Sources of Error

1. Hemolysis will modify the sedimentation rate.

2. Dirty tubes will cause inaccurate results; all traces of alcohol, ether, or acetone must be removed.
3. The exact concentration of anticoagulant is important. If it is higher than recommended, the ESR will be slowed down.
4. The tube must be placed in an upright position.
5. Bubbles in the tube will affect the sedimentation rate.
6. The temperature should remain between 20° and 27° C.
7. The test should be done within 2 hours of collection (or 12 hours if EDTA is used and the blood is stored at 4° C).

THE RETICULOCYTE COUNT

Red blood cells progress through a series of stages of development prior to reaching full maturity. The immature stages are confined to the bone marrow except for a small percentage of the cells in the stage just preceding the erythrocyte stage. This cell stage is termed the diffusely basophilic or reticulocyte stage. The reticulocyte spends approximately two days maturing in the bone marrow and is then released into the blood where it spends one more day maturing prior to becoming an erythrocyte.

Approximately 1 percent of the total circulating red cell population are reticulocytes. The reticulocyte count is significant in that it is an indication of effective red cell production in the bone marrow. The life-span of the normal red cell is approximately 120 days and the body normally replaces about 1 percent of the adult red cells every day. Increases or decreases in the number of circulating reticulocytes, therefore, indicate hyperplastic (active formation) or hypoplastic (underactive formation) bone marrow activity. The discovery of reticulocytosis may lead to discovering a hidden (occult) disease such as chronic hemorrhage or unrecognized hemolysis. Persistently low reticulocyte counts, accompanied by anemia, usually indicate defective erythropoiesis. Persistent absence of reticulocytes from peripheral blood in aplastic anemias usually indicates a poor prognosis. Persistently elevated reticulocyte counts accompany chronic hemolytic anemia; a drop to very low values indicates bone marrow failure.

In diseases such as aplastic anemia and other conditions where bone marrow production is decreased, the reticulocyte count will be below the normal 0.5% to 1.5%. In diseases such as thalassemia, hemolytic anemia, acute blood loss, and hyperactive adrenal glands, the production of red blood cells is increased and, therefore, the reticulocyte count will be increased above normal. In newborn infants, the percentage is 2.5% to 6.5%; this falls to adult range within a few weeks.

Reticulocyte counts should be corrected to reflect the total production of red cells, irrespective of the number (or concentration) of the red cells present in the blood sample. The formula for this correction follows:

$$\text{corrected reticulocyte count in \%} = \frac{\text{patient's hematocrit} \times \text{reticulocyte count in \%}}{\text{normal hematocrit of 42\% for women, 45\% for men}}$$

Equipment and Reagents

1. reticulocyte stain, any of the following:
   a. 1% saline solution of brilliant cresyl blue

b. 1% methyl alcohol solution of brilliant cresyl blue
c. new methylene blue N solution
   stains should be filtered just prior to use
2. glass slides
3. microhematocrit tubes, applicator sticks, or pasteur pipets
4. small test tubes (12 × 75 mm)
5. microscope
6. tally counters

Principle

Reticulocytes still retain a small amount of RNA and a few ribosomes, which disappear before the cells become mature. These substances cause the cells to appear polychromatophilic when stained with Wright's stain. These cells are called diffusely basophilic erythrocytes. Special stains, called supravital stains, are used to stain these cells in the living state. When exposed to the vital stains, the RNA and ribosomes form aggregates within the cells that take up the basic stain and appear as blue-black reticula or as blue-black dots.

Procedure

1. Put three drops of filtered stain in a small test tube.
2. Add three drops of well-mixed anticoagulated or capillary blood to the tube containing the stain.
3. Mix the contents of the tube thoroughly and allow the mixture to sit for 10-15 minutes. This time is necessary for the reticulocytes to take up the stain.
4. After 10-15 minutes have elapsed, remix the contents of the tube.
5. With a Pasteur pipet (or applicator sticks or microhematocrit tube), remove a drop of the blood-stain mixture and place it on a glass slide and make a blood smear. Make one or two additional smears.
6. Allow the smears to dry.
7. The smears may be counter-stained with Wright's stain, if desired. However, this step may be omitted as it is not necessary for the staining of the RNA and ribosomes.
8. Place the slide on the microscope stage. Using the 10× objective, locate an area of the smear where the red blood cells are evenly distributed and not overlapping each other. Add a drop of immersion oil to the slide and change to the 100× objective.
9. Locate an area where there are approximately 150 to 200 red cells per microscopic field.
10. Count the number of reticulocytes seen per 1000 red blood cells (mature red cells and reticulocytes). The reticulum will appear heavy in some cells and sparse in others, depending upon the maturity of the cells (Figure 36). Younger reticulocytes will display more RNA and ribosomes than the more mature reticulocytes. Using two tally counters will facilitate enumeration of the total red cell count with one counter and tally of the number of reticulocytes with the second counter. The slide is moved in the same manner as indicated for the

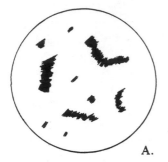 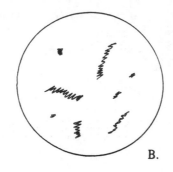 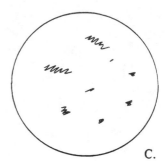

Figure 36. Reticula in reticulocytes showing stages of maturity.
(A) younger reticulocyte
(B) intermediate reticulocyte
(C) very mature reticulocyte

differential count until 1000 red cells have been counted and the
reticulocytes tallied.

11. A second count should be done using another slide from the same
blood sample. The two results should agree within ± 10% of each other.
If not, repeat the count on a third smear.

12. Average the two results and calculate the reticulocyte count as follows:

$$\% \ reticulocytes = \frac{number \ of \ reticulocytes \ counted \ in \ 1000 \ red \ cells}{1000 \ red \ cells \ (erythrocytes + reticulocytes)} \times 100$$

13. Calculation of the corrected reticulocyte count may be done.

Discussion

1. New methylene blue stain is generally preferred over brilliant cresyl
   blue because of the inconsistency of the staining properties of the
   latter.
2. There are several methods employed by laboratories in performing a
   reticulocyte count. All procedures are based on the same general
   principles as previously described. Some of these variations are listed
   below.
   a. The stain-blood mixture may be made in a microhematocrit tube,
      in a red cell pipet, or on a glass slide. The 1:1 ratio of stain to
      blood is usually retained, but this is not absolutely critical.
   b. The staining time may vary somewhat in different procedures.
      However, it should not be less than 10 minutes for good stain
      uptake.
3. The ratio of stain to blood should be altered in blood samples having
   either high or low hematocrits. Less stain should be added to samples
   having very low hematocrits, more stain to samples having very high
   hematocrits.
4. It is very important that the blood and stain be remixed before making
   the smears. Because reticulocytes have a lower specific gravity than
   mature red cells, they will settle on top of the red cells in the mixture.
5. For ease of counting, a glass ocular may be inserted into the eyepiece.

The ocular forms a large square on the field of view. The large square contains a smaller square that is 1/10 the area of the large square. The reticulocytes are counted in the large square, the red cells in the smaller square in successive fields. At least 300 red cells should be counted in the small square, providing an estimate of reticulocytes among 3000 red cells. The calculation is:

$$reticulocytes\ in\ \% = \frac{number\ of\ reticulocytes\ in\ large\ square \times 100}{number\ of\ red\ cells\ in\ small\ square \times 10}$$

6. Several red cell inclusions may be stained by the methylene blue and brilliant cresyl blue stains, in addition to RNA and ribosomes. Heinz bodies will stain a faint blue-green and usually appear at the periphery of the cell membrane. Howell-Jolly bodies stain deep blue-purple usually appear as several granules in a cluster and are most easily confused with reticulocytes. However, iron deposits and Howell-Jolly will be found in the same configuration on Wright-stained smears.

7. The margin or error in reticulocyte counts will vary. In the previously outlined procedure, range of error is expected to be ± 25% for normal reticulocyte counts. The margin or error becomes less as the reticulocyte count increases, however. Error is the result of random distribution of the reticulocytes among adult erythrocytes.

THE PLATELET COUNT

Platelets are formed in the bone marrow as the result of the selective fragmentation of the cytoplasm of a cell called the megakaryocyte. The platelet is then released into the peripheral blood and has a lifespan of approximately 8-12 days. Normally about one-third of the platelets are sequestered in the spleen. They are metabolically very active. They function in maintaining capillary integrity and in hemostasis (control of bleeding). They readily adhere to one another (aggregation) and readily attach to foreign surfaces (adhesion).

The readiness with which platelets aggregate and adhere necessitates special precautions during the collection of the blood specimen and the immediate addition of an anticoagulant. The use of EDTA helps to decrease the clumping of the platelets. Although capillary blood may be used, the results are generally less satisfactory and significantly lower than counts performed on venous blood.

The normal range for the platelet count is 150,000 to 400,000 per μl (0.15

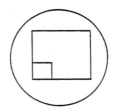

Figure 37. Eyepiece insert.

to 0.40 $\pm$ $10^{12}/1$). Increased platelet counts (thrombocytosis) may be found after splenectomy, in polycythemia vera, chronic myelogenous leukemia, idiopathic thrombocythemia, inflammatory reactions, acute posthemorrhagic anemia, and other myeloproliferative disorders. Low platelet counts (thrombocytopenia) may be found in aplastic disorders, immune thrombocytopenic purpuras, acute leukemias, pernicious anemia, following chemotherapy and radiation therapy, increased splenic sequestration of blood, and splenomegaly.

Platelet counts are of great importance in helping to diagnose bleeding disorders. However, the platelet count must be accompanied by additional platelet function studies and other coagulation tests before an accurate assessment of the bleeding antitheses can be established. Generally, bleeding episodes do not occur unless the platelet count is below 50,000/ μl (0.05 $\times$ $10^{12}/1$).

A number of direct methods for platelet counting have been proposed. The most reliable is that in which platelets are counted in a special phase hemocytometer using phase microscopy. This is the reference method for platelet counts. Electronic platelet counting yields satisfactory results that correlate well with the reference method. Adoption of electronic platelet counting should be based on a comparison of the instrument with the reference method.

The Rees-Ecker Method utilizes a standard hemocytometer and bright light microscope. An indirect method proposed by Fonio may be used but is less accurate than the direct procedures.

Rees-Ecker Method

The Rees-Ecker Method is included in this manual for the benefit of those laboratories without a phase microscope.

Equipment and Reagents

1. Rees-Ecker diluting fluid, which contains sodium citrate, formaldehyde, and brilliant cresyl blue. It is necessary to filter the Rees-Ecker solution just prior to using it in order to remove any precipitation of stain or other debris.
2. red cell pipets
3. hemocytometer and cover glass
4. petri dish with moist paper toweling or cotton swab
5. microscope

Principle

When the whole blood is mixed with the Rees-Ecker solution, the red cells and platelets are preserved and the platelets stained by the brilliant cresyl blue. The standard hemocytometer is filled and the platelets are counted. The count is checked by examining the platelets on the Wright's stained smear.

Procedure

1. Two red cell pipets are used. In each, the well-mixed anticoagulated

blood (or the second drop of capillary blood from a capillary puncture) is drawn exactly to the 0.5 mark and diluted to the 101 mark with the Rees-Ecker solution (1:200 dilution as with the red cell count). Rotate the pipet while filling to properly mix blood with the diluting solution.

2. Mix by shaking for 3-5 minutes. The count should be done within 30 minutes.
3. Discard the first 4-5 drops from the pipet.
4. Fill both sides of a scrupulously clean hemocytometer with the diluted blood. One side is filled with dilution from one pipet; the other side from the second dilution. (A red cell count may also be performed since the same dilution is made for each. This red count may then be used in checking the chamber platelet count by the indirect method of Fonio.)
5. The hemocytometer is placed under a dish cover (or in a petri dish) with a moist towel or cotton swab for 10-15 minutes. The moist toweling prevents evaporation of the fluid while the platelets are settling in the chamber.
6. Place the hemocytometer on the microscope stage and using the 10X objective, locate the center square millimeter area of the chamber (as with chamber red counts). Carefully change to the 40X objective and count the platelets in the 5 "R" squares on both sides of the counting chamber. Platelets are much smaller than the red cells. They are approximately $2\text{-}4\mu$ in diameter and appear as light blue round, oval, or slightly irregular refractile objects. There should be 3-8 platelets per section (R section). Take care not to confuse platelets with debris. Calculate the number of platelets in the average of the two counts.
7. Calculate the number of platelets per μl by the following method:

$$\begin{matrix} number\ of \\ platelets\ in \\ 1\ \mu l\ of \\ whole\ blood \end{matrix} = \begin{matrix} average\ number \\ of\ platelets\ counted \\ in\ the\ 5\ R \\ squares \end{matrix} \times \begin{matrix} dilution \\ correction \\ factor \\ (200) \end{matrix} \times \begin{matrix} volume \\ correction \\ factor \\ (50) \end{matrix}$$

Example:
An average of 30 platelets were counted in the 10 R squares.

$\begin{matrix} number\ of\ platelets \\ in\ 1\ \mu l\ of\ whole\ blood \end{matrix} = 30 \times 200 \times 50$

$number\ of\ platelets = 30 \times 10{,}000$

$number\ of\ platelets = 300{,}000/\mu l\ (0.3 \times 10^{12}/l)$

8. Check the platelet count by scanning the Wright-stained smear and estimating the number of platelets per field in ratio to the number of red cells per field. Reasonable agreement should be obtained or the platelet count should be repeated.

Discussion

1. If clumps of platelets are observed in the counting chamber, the procedure must be repeated. Clumping is due to poor technique in

blood collection or to inadequate mixing of the blood.

2. It is of utmost importance that the pipets are clean and the diluting fluid is freshly filtered. It is equally important that the hemocytometer be thoroughly cleaned prior to filling the chambers.

3 As in red and white counts, the platelets should be evenly distributed in the chamber.

4. If the platelet count is extremely low or extremely high, altering the dilution will increase the accuracy of the count. Dilute low counts 1:100; dilute high counts 1:500.

5. The margin of error for the platelet count is estimated to be $\pm$ 15-25%.

Becker-Cronkite Method

This method employs the use of a phase microscope, which enables the platelets to be identified not only on the basis of their size and shape but also on their structure.

Principle

Whole anticoagulated blood (preferably) is diluted with 1% ammonium oxalate, which hemolyzes the red cells. The platelets are then counted using the phase hemocytometer and phase microscope. The count is then checked by examining the blood smear.

Equipment and Reagents

1. 1% ammonium oxalate, which must be filtered just prior to use
2. red cell pipets
3. phase hemocytometer with a thin No. 1 or 1½ coverslip
4. petri dish with moist filter paper or cotton gauze swab
5. phase microscope

Procedure

The step-by-step procedure will not be discussed here since much of the preliminary procedure is very similar to the Rees-Ecker procedure.

1. EDTA anticoagulated blood is preferred. Plastic or siliconized syringes and test tubes may be preferable, but Vacutainer tubes are satisfactory. The well-mixed blood is diluted in the red cell pipet (1:200 dilution) with 1% ammonium oxalate. Two pipets are prepared.

2. The mixture is shaken, and phase hemocytometer is filled, placed under the petri dish cover with the moist paper, and allowed to settle for 10-15 minutes.

3. The hemocytometer is placed on the microscope stage and the platelets are counted using the 43× phase objective. The same areas are counted as in the regular counting chamber. The background will appear black, with the white cells, platelets, debris and lines of the hemocytometer being illuminated. The platelets have a light purple sheen. Debris and dirt will be distinguished by the high amount of refraction. Calculate the averaged platelet counts done on each side of the chamber.

4. Calculate the platelet count by the same formula used for the calculation of the red cell count or the Rees-Ecker platelet count.

Discussion

1. The same items discussed in the Rees-Ecker method also apply to the phase contrast procedure.
2. The dilution of the blood with 1% ammonium oxalate is more stable than blood diluted with Rees-Ecker fluid. With 1% ammonium oxalate, the dilution is stable for at least 8 hours.
3. Once the technologist is experienced, the margin of error using phase microscopy can be maintained at less than 10%.

Fonio Indirect Method

Equipment and Reagents

1. magnesium sulfate solution (14%)
2. glass slides
3. red cell pipet
4. red cell diluting fluid
5. applicator sticks (if anticoagulated blood is used)
6. hemocytometer with cover glass
7. Wright's stain
8. microscope

Principle

The ratio of platelets to red cells is determined by counting the platelets on a blood smear. The red count is performed on the hemocytometer and multiplied by the platelet-to-red-cell-ratio.

Procedure

1. Using the applicator stick, place a drop of well-mixed anticoagulated blood on the slide and make a blood smear. Allow smear to air dry.
2. Using the red cell pipet, prepare a 1:200 dilution (draw blood to 0.5 mark and dilute to 101 mark) of the well-mixed anticoagulated blood with 14% magnesium sulfate. Mix 3 minutes.
3. If capillary blood is to be used, the 14% magnesium sulfate is placed on the cleansed finger (toe, heel, etc.) and the puncture is made through the magnesium sulfate solution. This prevents clumping of the platelets. A blood smear and a red cell dilution are then made.
4. Stain the smear.
5. Perform a red cell count on the hemocytometer.
6. On the stained blood smear, count 1000 red cells using the oil immersion objective. Record the number of platelets seen during the count. (A paper window may be inserted into the eyepiece of the microscope, which will facilitate easier counting of the red cells.) Calculate the platelet count.
7. Calculation of the number of platelets per μl is as follows:

$$\text{number of platelets per }\mu l \text{ of whole blood} = \frac{\text{number of platelets counted on blood smear}}{\text{number of red cells counted on blood smear}} \times \text{red cell count (by hemocytometer)}$$

Example:

    Platelets counted on smear   = 60
    RBC counted on smear   = 1000
    RBC count on hemocytometer   = 4,000,000/µl (4.0 × 10¹²/l)

$$\frac{\text{platelet count}}{\text{per }\mu l \text{ blood}} = \frac{50}{1000} \times 4,000,000$$

$$\text{platelet count} = \frac{1}{20} \times 4,000,000$$

$$\text{platelet count} = 200,000/\mu l \ (0.20 \times 10^{12}/l)$$

Discussion

1. The indirect method gives higher values than the direct methods and is less accurate. It is not widely used, but may be used as a check on the direct count.
2. When counting the red blood cells on the blood smear, the count should be performed in an area where the red cells are evenly distributed and not over lapping (150-200 cells per field).
3. The pattern of counting is the same as for differentials and reticulocyte counting.
4. Extreme care should be taken when making the smear in order that the platelets will not be clumped. If clumping is present, a new smear should be made.

STUDY QUESTIONS

1. List the normal values for the sedimentation rate for the following:

    Wintrob Method   *Westergren Method*
    Men   _____   Men   _____
    Women   _____   Women   _____
    Children _____   Children _____

2. Indicate whether the sedimentation rate is increased or decreased by the following:
    a. temperature at 4°C
    b. delay of 3 hours (in double oxalate)
    c. microcytic erythrocytes
    d. increased plasma proteins
    e. dehydration
    f. anemia
    g. infection
    h. 1:5 dilution of blood with liquid anticoagulant
    i. 13 × 100 mm test tube rather than usual sedimentation tube
    j. polycythemia
3. The factor that affects the sedimentation rate the most is _____
4. Define:
    a. viscosity

b. density

5. Explain why a blood sample having a high hematocrit will have a low sedimentation rate.

6. The sedimentation rate is (directly, inversely) proportional to the number of plasma proteins in the blood sample.

7. List three purposes for performing the sedimentation rate.

· 8. The sedimentation rate is (directly, inversely) proportional to the density of the blood sample.

9. The sedimentation rate is (directly, inversely) proportional to the viscosity of the blood sample.

10. Following I.V. fluid therapy, the sedimentation rate would probably be (increased, decreased). Why?

11. What are the three stages in the sedimentation of red cells?

12. New methylene blue stain is an example of a _____ stain.

13. The substances that form aggregates in the reticulocyte during staining with new methylene blue are _____ and _____.

14. The reticulocytes' counterpart on a Wright's stained blood smear is called _____.

15. What is the significance of reticulocyte count?

16. The normal reticulocyte count is _____.

17. Indicate whether the reticulocyte count will be increased or decreased in the following:
   a. hemolytic anemia
   b. aplastic anemia
   c. hemorrhage
   d. hyperactive adrenal glands

18. Give the formula for calculating the reticulocyte count.

19. The ratio of blood to reticulocyte stain is usually _____.

20. Describe the procedure for performing the reticulocyte count.

21. An alternative to new methylene blue stain for reticulocyte counting is _____.

22. The _____ objective is used to perform the reticulocyte count.

23. The normal range for platelets is _____.

24. Give three methods for performing platelet counts.

25. Bleeding episodes will probably not occur unless the platelet count is below _____.

26. Average platelet size is _____.

27. The proper dilution for hemocytometer platelet counting is _____

28. What are the purposes of placing the filled hemocytometer under the petri dish cover with the wet gauze sponge?

29. Platelets are cytoplasmic fragments of _____.

30. List four disorders in which the platelet count may be increased.

31. List three disorders in which the platelet count is decreased.

32. What type of stain is contained in the Rees-Ecker solution?

33. Give the formula for calculating the platelet count by hemocytometry.

34. The _____ objective is used to perform platelet counts.

35. The reliability of the chamber platelet counts may be checked by examining the _____.

36. Briefly describe the Fonio indirect method of platelet counting.

Chapter 8

COAGULATION AND HEMOSTASIS

OBJECTIVES

The student will learn and/or identify:

1. The complex interaction of platelets, blood vessels, and coagulation proteins necessary for hemostasis.
2. the three platelet activities that occur in the formation of a platelet thrombus: adhesion, aggregation, and release of vasoactive substances.
3. the conditions or circumstances that can lead to the activation of the coagulation process.
4. the coagulation proteins.
5. the prothrombin, fibrinogen, contact, and kinin families of coagulation proteins.
6. thrombin as the enzyme produced by the interaction of the coagulation substances.
7. the two systems of coagulation: the extrinsic and intrinsic systems.
8. the relationship of the kinin system to coagulation.
9. the chemical effect that thrombin exerts on fibrinogen to produce fibrin.
10. the importance of factor XIII in hemostasis.
11. the various coagulation tests that identify abnormalities in the coagulation process.
12. the two types of anticoagulant therapy used today.
13. the anticoagulant activities of the two types of drugs and indicate the tests used to monitor the effectiveness of these activities.

INTRODUCTION

Blood coagulation is now understood to be a molecular process regulated by a delicate interaction of three systems: coagulation and fibrinolytic proteins, platelets, and the endothelium of blood vessels. When there is injury to a blood vessel, the process begins that will eventually stop the escape of blood from the vessel and repair the damage that the vessel has received. The process of arresting the flow of blood is called hemostasis. There are many aspects of hemostasis, one of which is the process of coagulation.

In order that normal hemostasis can be achieved, three highly complex mechanisms must be functioning properly. These three mechanisms are (1) the blood vessels, (2) blood platelets, and (3) blood coagulation and fibrinolytic substances. The most immediate response to vessel damage is the response of platelets that adhere to vessel walls, aggregate together, and release vasoactive substances during their process of forming a white thrombus, a platelet plug. The release of vasoactive substances causes constriction of the damaged blood vessel, thus reducing the blood flow through the vessel. The response of the blood vessel to the vasoconstrictor (serotonin) is therefore important in the hemostatic process, as are the platelets in plug formation and release of vasoactive substances. The coagulation substances, representing part of the third component in hemostasis, interact to create a fibrin network that solidifies and supports the platelet thrombus. Ultimately there is slow lysis of the clot by the fibrinolytic proteins and final repair of the injured site. Closely associated with the entire process is a fourth system, the kinin system, which will be briefly discussed in the cascade mechanism.

A basic knowledge of the various aspects of hemostasis is necessary to understanding the laboratory coagulation procedures.

COAGULATION

The formation of the fibrin stands in coagulation is facilitated by the complex interaction of eleven substances, called the coagulation factors. Ten of these substances are normally found in plasma, the eleventh is extrinsic to the vascular system. Most of these substances exist in their inactive form until they are activated by some mechanism. These factors have been given Roman numeral classification due to the confusion that existed a few years ago when each factor was identified by several names. Table I lists these factors along with their more commonly used names.

The actual interaction of these substances in the formation of fibrin cannot be known for certain because blood behaves differently in vivo. For

TABLE I

Factor	Name
I	Fibrinogen
II	Prothrombin
III	Tissue Thromboplastin, Thrombokinase
IV	Calcium
V	Labile Factor, Proaccelerin
VII	Stable Factor, Proconvertin
VIII	Antihemophilic Factor, Antihemophilic A Factor Antihemophilic Globulin
IX	Christmas Factor, Antihemophilic B Factor Plasma Thromboplastin Component
X	Stuart-Power Factor, Stuart Factor
XI	Plasma Thromboplastin Antecedent (PTA)
XII	Contact Factor, Hageman Factor
XIII	Fibrin Stabilizing Factor, Fibrinose

purposes of understanding the in vitro process, the researchers have divided the coagulation process into two systems, the *extrinsic system* and the *intrinsic system*. All substances required for the formation of fibrin via the intrinsic pathway are located in the blood. The extrinsic pathway requires factor III, tissue thromboplastin, which is released into the vascular system by damaged tissues. The interaction of the coagulation substances at certain stages of the coagulation process requires a platelet phospholipid, called platelet factor 3 (PF-3), which is released from platelets during platelet thrombus formation. Although the systems are divided for purpose of laboratory evaluation, it is most probable that tissue thromboplastin activates both systems in vivo. Coagulation through the extrinsic pathway is very rapid; only 10-12 seconds are required for clotting, while approximately 1.5 minutes are needed for clotting to occur in the intrinsic system. Figure 38 schematically portrays the interaction of the coagulation factors in the "cascading" 2-system process of fibrin formation. The activated forms of the coagulation proteins are proteolytic enzymes which, as indicated in Figure 38, alter the inactive forms of their substrates and change them to active forms.

The coagulation process can be activated by several mechanisms and/or substances. When the blood vessel is damaged, the exposure of the vascular endothelium is a potent activation mechanism. The release of tissue thromboplastin results in rapid fibrin deposition at the site of injury. Any wettable surface, i.e. glass, triggers the activation of factor XII. Kaolin and allegic acid are employed as activators in commercial laboratory reagents. Antigen-antibody complexes, platelet surfaces, and kallikrein are additional activating substances.

THE COAGULATION FACTORS

The Coagulation factors may be divided into four groups based on their properties and activities. The *Fibrinogen family* consists of factors I, VIII, V, and XIII. They are high molecular weight glycoproteins that are consumed during coagulation. They are, therefore, present in plasma and absent in serum. Factors V and VIII are extremely heat labile and are easily destroyed by prolonged in vitro incubation. The fibrinogen family factors are not absorbed by barium sulfate.

The *Prothrombin family* includes factors II, VII, IX, and X. These factors are low molecular weight glycoproteins. Vitamin K is required for their syntheses in the liver. Coumarin drugs inhibit Vitamin K syntheses of these proteins, resulting in metabolically inactive proteins being produced. Factors VII, IX, and X are not consumed during coagulation and are, therefore, found in plasma and serum. All four factors are stable and thus found in stored plasma. All four factors are absorbed by barium sulfate.

The *Contact Family* is composed of factors XII and XI. Factor XII is activated by various substances to initiate the clotting process. Factors XII and XI are not consumed during coagulation, are not absorbed by barium sulfate, and are relatively stable. They are present in serum and plasma.

The *Kinin family* includes prekallikrein (Fletcher Factor), kallikrein, high molecular weight (HMW) kininogen (Fitzgerald Factor), and brady-kinin. Some of these substances are intricately involved in the activation of

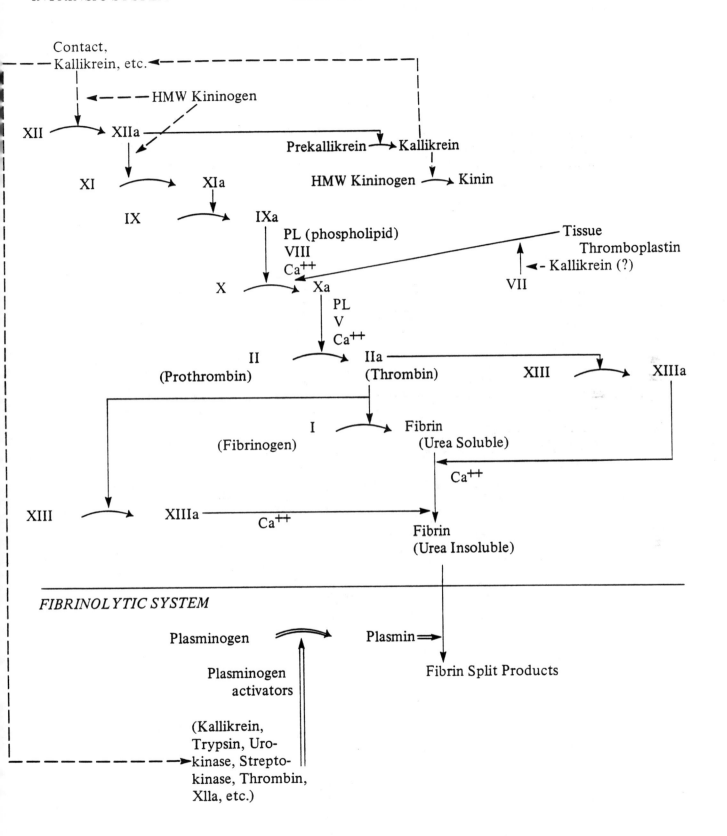

Figure 38.

several (?) of the coagulation and fibrinolytic proteins. Vascular permeability is increased by bradykinin. The reader is urged to consult a reliable hematology reference book for a detailed description of each of the proteins discussed.

The interaction of the factors, whatever the mechanism, is necessary to produce an enzymatic substance that does *not* normally exist in the vascular system. This substance is thrombin. Thrombin is necessary to alter fibrinogen (Factor I) molecules to form fibrin monomers, which in turn form fibrin. Fibrinogen is a large globular protein composed of three polypeptide chains, named α, β, and γ. Thrombin attacks the arginine-glycine bonds of α and β polypeptide chains and cleaves four small portions from the ends of these two chains. These four small cleaved segments are called fibrinopeptides. The large portion of the fibrinogen molecule remaining is called a fibrin monomer. Many monomers are formed and these form side-to-side and end-to-end linkages through hydrogen bonds, and fibrin is formed. This first-formed fibrin is flaccid, unstable, quickly dissolved by 5M urea, and is termed urea-soluble fibrin. The activated form of factor XIII (a transamindase) and calcium ions convert the hydrogen bonds of urea-soluble fibrin to covalent bonds creating firm, stable, urea insoluble fibrin. (Figure 39)

The fibrin strands are formed on the surface of the platelet due to the fact that many coagulation factors have absorbed onto the platelet membrane. Thus the fibrin network stabilizes the already formed platelet plug. The proteins actin and myosin in the platelets further strengthen the plug. Refer to Chapter 7 for additional information on platelets.

There are limiting mechanisms of hemostasis and coagulation. If coagulation occurred spontaneously, the individual would be subjected to

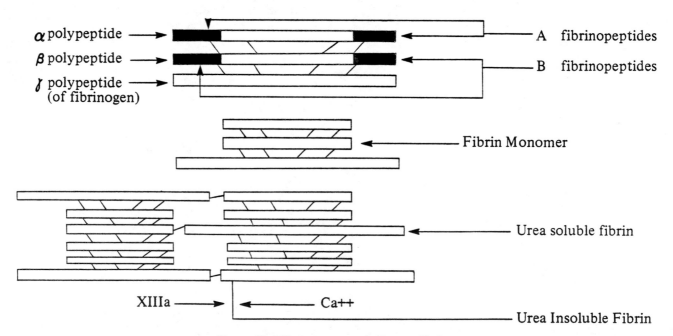

Figure 39. Fibrinogen conversion to fibrin.

life-threatening circumstances of vessel occlusion, organ failure, ultimately shock and death. Antithrombins, platelet inhibitors, and other inactivators are in the vascular system. These substances help to maintain the fluidity of the blood under normal circumstances.

When injury occurs and coagulation takes place, it is extremely important that the thrombus remain localized at the site of the injury. Several circumstances are present that keep the clot localized: (1) coagulation activators are not normally present in the blood; (2) when injury occurs, platelets accumulate at the site, bringing absorbed coagulation factors, which then become activated, and fibrin is formed on their surfaces. Any activating substances that do manage to escape into the circulating blood are quickly degraded by the liver or inactivated by inhibitors or inactivators; (3) fibrinolysis (fibrin dissolution) is activated when coagulation begins. Clot lysis soon restores circulation to the area.

COAGULATION SCREENING PROCEDURES

Deficiencies in the coagulation processes may cause a variety of bleeding disorders, from asymptomatic to severe. Several tests may be performed before the abnormality is fully identified. A series of tests, called a coagulation screen, coagulation work-up, or coagulation panel are those routine tests performed to detect deficiencies and abnormalities. A good coagulation screen should include tests designed to detect the largest majority of coagulation abnormalities. A good set of screening tests should include bleeding time, coagulation time, clot retraction, prothrombin time, activated partial thromboplastin time, and platelet count.

The bleeding time, clot retraction, and platelet count should detect most platelet abnormalities. The activated partial thromboplastin time will detect deficiencies in the intrinsic coagulation system. The prothrombin time will detect deficiencies in the extrinsic coagulation system. The coagulation time will provide another method for assessing the interaction of platelets and the coagulation factors.

If a coagulation abnormality is discovered from the results of the coagulation work-up, the exact deficiency or disorder should be identified. Factor identification studies should be performed if the prothrombin time and/or activated partial thromboplastin time are found to be abnormal. Once the actual factor deficiency is identified, then a factor assay should be performed to determine the concentration of the deficient factor (or factors). Platelet abnormalities should be followed up with adhesion, aggregation, factor-3 availability, and prothrombin consumption studies to determine the actual platelet disorder.

In contrast to the coagulation disorders that cause bleeding problems, there are those disorders of coagulation in which coagulation occurs without evidence of injury; that is, thrombus formation that occludes vessels and poses life-threatening circumstances for the victims, i.e. coronary thrombosis, cerebrovascular accident, etc. In order to reduce the likelihood of further thrombotic episodes in these individuals, anticoagulant therapy is given. Monitoring the effects of drugs that are to be given is important. The coagulation time must not be so reduced as to create a bleeding episode, yet it must be reduced sufficiently to prevent further thrombosis. Coumarin drugs and heparin are the two kinds of anticoagulant therapy most generally used today.

The coumarins inhibit synthesis of factors II, VII, IX, X, thus reducing the concentration of these four coagulation proteins, which in turn reduces the likelihood of thrombus formation. The prothrombin time is generally used to monitor coumarin therapy since all except IX are found in the extrinsic coagulation pathway. The activated partial thromboplastin time may be used to monitor heparin therapy. Heparin (together with antithrombin III) inhibits thrombin from attacking fibrinogen molecules, thus inhibiting fibrin formation. Heparin has inhibitory effects on some of the coagulation factors as well. The Lee-White Clotting Time is sometimes used to monitor heparin therapy, but it is *not* recommended due to the wide variability in techniques and procedures.

Recent advances in monitoring anticoagulant therapy using synthetic fluorogenic or chromogenic substrates have been introduced, which will play key roles in the development of diagnostic methodologies to test hemostatic function in the future. Antithrombin III determination has already become a routine diagnostic test in major medical centers throughout the United States and Europe. Perhaps the entire battery of coagulation tests in the future will involve fluorometric or chromogenic analyses of the concentration of activated forms of many coagulation and fibrinolytic proteins.

ACCURACY OF COAGULATION TESTS

Accuracy in performing coagulation studies is dependent upon several conditions. Some of these precautions will be discussed. All technologists should endeavor to keep in mind these important aspects of quality control in coagulation studies.

1. Only good quality glassware should be used. It should be borosilicate type I glass, not soda lime glass. It should not be reused and care should be taken to keep it stored in a clean, dust-free area. Glassware that has been washed may have a residual detergent, mercury, or dirt that could prolong coagulation tests.
2. Proper temperature (37°C) is *absolutely necessary*. One of the three critical aspects of enzyme studies is temperature control.
3. Incubation time is also critical in coagulation studies. The heat labile factors V and VIII are quickly destroyed by prolonged incubation. Enzymes are also easily destroyed by excessive heating.
4. The type of anticoagulant used is important. Depending upon the procedure or reagents used in the studies, one should always use the anticoagulant indicated in the procedure. The control plasmas should also contain the same anticoagulant as that used in the collected blood sample.
5. Reaction time is extremely important. Most procedures are timed within one-tenth of a second, so starting and stopping the stopwatch or instrument must be accurately done.
6. The plasma must be removed from the red cells as quickly as possible.

Centrifugation and removal of the plasma must be done *within 30 minutes of collection*. The plasma may be refrigerated or placed on ice after being removed from the cells. The tests should then be performed as soon as possible.

7. Hemolyzed plasma should *never* be used for coagulation studies. Phospholipids from red cell membranes will accelerate the clotting times.

8. Normal and abnormal control plasma must be used on a daily basis to determine the accuracy of the test results. These plasmas are available from several manufacturers of laboratory reagents.

9. Refer to Chapter 10 for additional information on quality control in coagulation.

STUDY QUESTIONS

1. Coagulation of blood occurs as a result of the complex interaction of _____, _____, and _____.

2. Normally vessels _____ following injury, thus decreasing the blood flow.

3. The complete process of arresting the flow of blood from a vessel is called _____.

4. List three activities of platelets during the formation of the platelet thrombus.

5. Platelets provide _____, which is necessary for the clotting of blood.

6. The two systems of in vitro coagulation are _____ and _____.

7. List 5 substances that can activate the coagulation process.

8. There are _____ coagulation factors; _____ of these factors are proteins; _____ is calcium.

9. _____ is the only extrinsic coagulation factor.

10. There are _____ families, or groups, of coagulation proteins.
   a. Name the families.
   b. Indicate the factors that belong to each group.
   c. Describe the characteristics of each group.
   d. Which factors are vitamin K dependent?

11. The enzymatic substance necessary for the formation of fibrin is produced by the interactions of the coagulation factors. This substance is called _____.

12. The precursor of thrombin is _____.

13. Diagram the two systems of coagulation.

14. Coagulation factor _____ is called the fibrin stabilizing factor.

15. How does thrombin act upon fibrinogen to form fibrin?

16. Describe the effect that XIII has upon fibrin.

17. Activated XIII is a _____ (type of enzyme).

18. Platelets contain _____ and _____ that are necessary for clot retraction.

19. Substances that prevent spontaneous coagulation in vivo are called _____

20. What tests are useful in detecting platelet abnormalities?
21. Abnormalities of the intrinsic system are detected by employing the _____ test.
22. Extrinsic system abnormalities may be detected by the _____ test.
23. _____ studies are done to determine the specific coagulation factor that is deficient.
24. List additional platelet studies that are performed when platelet abnormalities are detected.
25. A _____ is performed to determine the concentration of a coagulation factor.
26. Two types of anticoagulant drugs used for therapeutic purposes are _____ and _____
27. Describe the anticoagulant activities of heparin.
28. Describe the anticoagulant activities of coumarin drugs.
29. Indicate the tests used to monitor the effects of the following anticoagulants given as therapy:
    a. heparin _____
    b. coumarin _____

COAGULATION TESTS

OBJECTIVES

The student will learn and/or define the following:

1. bleeding time.
2. coagulation time.
3. the normal values of the various coagulation tests performed in Chapter 9.
4. the significance of each test performed and why similar tests yield different normal values.
5. measures that will assure quality control in coagulation studies.
6. the reagents used in the coagulation tests included in this chapter.
7. the purpose of each reagent in objective #6.
8. the procedures for performing the various coagulation tests.
9. the procedure for performing factor identification studies.
10. the factors in the serum and plasma reagents used in identification studies.
11. the procedures for performing platelet function tests.
12. the significance of platelet function tests.
13. the variables that affect platelet function tests.

INTRODUCTION

The procedures used to study the various substances involved in the coagulation process have contributed much to the understanding of hemostasis. Many of the procedures are simple, reliable, and can be performed within a relatively short time. There are many procedures that are highly specialized, technically difficult, and impractical in all but the high volume or specialized research laboratores. Each laboratory should select a few procedures that will serve the diagnostic and therapeutic needs of that laboratory. This chapter will include a limited number of procedures that will serve to provide a responsible battery of coagulation tests, which will meet the needs of most laboratories.

The procedures included are simple but the utmost attention to technique is required to obtain reliable results. The procedures must be followed precisely each time if duplication of results is to be obtained. Modification of procedures or techniques *must be avoided*.

The procedures may be performed manually; some may be performed by semiautomated or completely automated methods. Some instruments detect the formation of a fibrin clot by the change in optical density of the plasma, others by interference of the electronic circuitry of the instrument when the clot forms. It is still essential to do both manual and automated procedures to learn the sources of error in the systems and to be prepared in the event of instrument malfunction.

BLEEDING TIME

The bleeding time is the time it takes platelets to form a platelet thrombus, which is supported by the vessel and fibrin network. It is dependent upon capillary function, platelets, and how efficiently tissue fluid accelerates the clotting process. The most important measures of the bleeding time, however, are platelet numbers and function. Prolonged bleeding will occur when the platelet count is below approximately 50,000 per μl and when there is platelet dysfunction (defective adhesion or aggregation).

Two methods of performing the bleeding time are the Duke method and the Ivy method. The Mielke template procedure, which is a variation of the Ivy method, is recommended over both procedures because of its degree of standardization.

Duke Method

The duration of bleeding from a standard puncture wound is measured. The length of time depends upon the function of platelets and the integrity of the vessel wall. Normal time is up to 6 minutes.

Equipment and Reagents

1. stopwatch with second hand
2. filter paper
3. sterile, disposable lancet
4. alcohol swabs or sponges

Procedure

1. Cleanse the ear lobe with the alcohol sponge and allow to dry.
2. Make a puncture with the sterile lancet, starting the stopwatch immediately. Make sure the puncture is deep enough to cause blood to appear. (A glass slide may be placed behind the ear to furnish support while making the puncture).
3. Blot the blood every 30 seconds with the filter paper. The filter paper should not touch the ear lobe.
4. When the bleeding ceases, stop the stopwatch, and record the bleeding time.

Discussion

1. Prolonged bleeding times should be repeated using the Ivy or Mielke procedure. Greater standardization of the length and depth of incision

and the constant pressure exerted on the blood vessels will give a more accurate measure of the bleeding time when these methods are used.

2. In small children, the heel may be used as the puncture site.
3. The puncture should be standardized as much as possible. Variations in the bleeding time result if the depth of the puncture is not sufficient to insure a free flow of blood.

Ivy Method

A pressure cuff is placed on the upper arm and inflated to 40 mm of mercury. A standardized puncture of the forearm is made, and the lenth of time required for bleeding to stop is recorded. Normal time is 2-7 minutes.

Equipment and Reagents

1. stopwatch with second hand
2. filter paper
3. a sterile, disposable lancet, capable of making a puncture 1 mm deep and 3 mm wide
4. alcohol swabs or sponges
5. blood pressure apparatus

Procedure

1. Place the pressure cuff on the upper part of the arm (above the elbow). Inflate the cuff to 40 mm of mercury and set the appartus to hold at this pressure.
2. Cleanse an area on the inner surface of the arm below the elbow with the alcohol sponge and allow to dry.
3. Grasping the under side of the arm firmly, pull the skin tightly. Make a puncture 3 mm wide, avoiding any veins. Start the stopwatch.
4. Blot the blood with the filter paper every 30 seconds. Take care not to touch the wound with the filter paper.
5. When bleeding ceases, stop the stop watch, and release the pressure cuff.
6. Record the bleeding time.

Discussion

1. The accuracy of this test may be increased by performing 2 or 3 tests and taking the average. A different area, of course, should be used for each puncture.
2. Bleeding times longer than 15 minutes should be repeated, using the other arm. The Mielke template procedure would give a more accurate result because of the ability to standardize the size of the incision.
3. The greatest source of variation in the Ivy test is standardization of the puncture. Where the bleeding time is less than 1 minute or greater than 7 minutes, the procedure should be repeated using the other arm.

Mielke Templete Variation of the Ivy Method

In this procedure, a sterile lancet is placed in a special handle capable of regulating the depth of incision to 1 mm. In addition, a rectangular polystyreen template that contains a slit 9 mm long is employed. Use of these two objects standardizes the length and depth of the puncture during the procedure. The same steps as described for the Ivy bleeding time are employed, utilizing the blood pressure apparatus. Normal values for this procedure are 2.5-10 minutes.

Although this procedure is the most accurate one used to determine the bleeding time, it may not be used routinely because of the small scars that result.

WHOLE BLOOD CLOTTING TIME

The coagulation time is the time it takes for blood to clot. Platelets and possibly all coagulation factors are measured. There are several methods for performing the whole blood clotting time, using either the capillary method or venous blood methods. Capillary methods have shorter times than the venous methods because tissue thromboplastin mixes with the blood during the puncture process, thus accelerating coagulation. In the venous methods, the blood is drawn from the vein; there is little opportunity for tissue thromboplastin to mix with the blood. Hence, the coagulation time is relatively long. Exposure of blood to a foreign surface initiates the clotting process.

Capillary Tube Method

A puncture of the finger is made and the blood is collected in two plain capillary tubes. A stopwatch is started prior to filling the tubes. The filled tubes are allowed to sit for a short period of time. At intervals of 30 seconds, the tubes are broken until a fibrin strand is seen between the two pieces of capillary tubes. The coagulation time is the time that elapsed between the production of the large drop of blood and the appearance of the fibrin. Normal values are 2-6 minutes.

Equipment and Reagents

1. stopwatch with a second hand
2. sterile, disposable lancet
3. alcohol swabs or sponges
4. plain capillary tubes (small tubes that contain no anticoagulant)

Procedure

1. Cleanse the finger with the alcohol sponge and allow to dry.
2. Make a relatively deep puncture with the sterile lancet. Wipe away the first drop of blood that appears.
3. Gently massage the finger to produce a large drop of blood, starting the stopwatch when this drop of blood appears. *Do not squeeze the finger, however.*
4. Fill two plain capillary tubes with the blood. Additional blood may be needed. If so, repeat the massaging process to produce additional drops of blood until the tubes are filled.

5. Place the capillary tubes on the table and allow 2 minutes to elapse. Make a note of which capillary tube was filled first and which end was filled first.
6. After 2 minutes, and at 30 second intervals thereafter, carefully break the capillary tubes with both hands. Start on the capillary tube which was filled first and at the end filled first. *Be careful not to pull the broken ends too far apart.* Look for a thread-like strand of fibrin between the two broken ends.
7. When the fibrin is seen, stop the stopwatch and record the coagulation time.

Discussion

1. Care should be taken when massaging the finger not to squeeze so firmly as to cause excessive mixing of tissue thromboplastin with the blood. This would shorten the coagulation time.
2. In order to ensure completion of the test in case the coagulation time is prolonged or not enough blood was collected, you may allow 3 minutes to elapse before breaking the tube the first time.
3. Hold the capillary tube downward while filling it. Fill the tubes to approximately three-fourths full.
4. The capillary tube method is a rapid screening procedure used primarily in the pre-surgical coagulation workup.
5. The capillary method has been discontinued in many laboratories because of the danger of contracting hepatitis from cuts obtained when breaking the tubes.

Lee and White Method

There are a number of modifications of the Lee-White procedure. They are all based on the same principle, however, and they all employ basically the same techniques. The size of the tubes, the amount of blood used, and the temperature at which the tests are done are the main variations in the modifications. Because of the degree of variation in technique, the Lee and White method should not be used to monitor heparin therapy.

The coagulation time of whole blood by the Lee-White Method is the length of time required for a measured amount of blood to clot under certain specified conditions. Venous blood is drawn, the stopwatch started when the blood enters the syringe, the blood placed into 3 test tubes, the tubes incubated at 37°C, and the tubes tilted at intervals until coagulation takes place. The coagulation time is recorded as the time from the point at which the blood first entered the syringe to the time at which the blood was clotted in tube number 3. The normal values are 5-15 minutes.

Equipment and Reagents

1. stopwatch with second hand
2. glass test tubes, 13 × 100 mm
3. water bath, 37°C
4. syringe (10 ml) and 20 gauge needle

Procedure

1. Three 13 × 100 mm test tubes are labelled no. 1, no. 2, no. 3.
2. Perform a venipuncture, using the 20 gauge needle, and withdraw 4 ml of blood. Start the stopwatch at the point when the blood enters the syringe.
3. Remove the needle from the syringe after collecting the blood. Carefully place 1 ml of the blood in test tube no. 3, 1 ml in tube no. 2, and 1 ml in tube no. 1. Discard the remaining blood.
4. Place the tubes in the 37°C water bath.
5. Allow 5 minutes to elapse, then gently tilt tube no. 1 to a 45° angle. Repeat the tilting procedure every 30 seconds until a clot has formed and blood will not spill out of the tube. Record the time it took the blood in tube no. 1 to clot.
6. Thirty seconds after tube no. 1 has clotted, tilt tube no. 2 and repeat step 5 until a clot is formed in tube no. 2. Record the results. Repeat this procedure for tube no. 3.
7. The coagulation time is reported as the time it took the blood in tube no. 3 to clot. Handling and tilting speed up coagulation so the time required for the blood to clot in tube no. 3 is a more accurate measure of the coagulation time of the blood sample.

Discussion

1. Care must be taken in performing the venipuncture in order to obtain a specimen that is not mixed with tissue thromboplastin nor hemolyzed. The blood should be drawn slowly so that no air bubbles enter the syringe. The blood should be handled gently when placing it in the test tubes because unnecessary agitation will shorten the coagulation time.
2. Exactly 1 ml of blood should be placed in each tube. Larger amounts increase the clotting time while smaller amounts shorten the clotting time.
3. The temperature of the water bath must be constant at 37°C. Fluctuations or higher or lower temperatures will affect the length of clotting time. In procedures that call for room temperature incubation of the test, the same precautions should be observed.
4. A modified method of the previous procedure, which is more sensitive to coagulation deficiencies, employs the use of siliconized glass test tubes in place of plain glass tubes. The clotting time, using the siliconized tubes and tilting them every five minutes, is 20-60 minutes. This procedure is not practical for routine coagulation screening due to the length of time involved.
5. One of the tubes can be left in the water bath and checked for clot retraction. Leaving the tube in the bath overnight will reveal any abnormal lysis of the clot.
6. The Lee-White has been most generally used to monitor heparin anti-coagulant therapy, but it is rapidly being replaced by the less variable activated partial thromboplastin time (APTT) in many laboratories.

CLOT RETRACTION

When the coagulation of blood is complete, the clot will begin to undergo contraction. Serum is expressed from the clot, and the clot becomes more compact. Clot retraction is dependent upon the function and number of platelets in the blood. Platelets contain two contractile proteins, actin and myosin, which are responsible for clot retraction (Thrombasthenin was the former name given to these two proteins.) If the platelet count is below 50,000 per μl or if platelet release of these proteins is abnormal, poor clot retraction can occur. Normally clot retraction is evident within 1-2 hours from the time the blood was drawn and should be complete within 24 hours. Whole fresh blood is placed in 37°C water bath, and examined at 1, 2, 4, and 24 hours for clot retraction.

Equipment and Reagents

1. water bath, 37°C
2. glass test tubes, 13 × 100 mm

Procedure

1. Perform a venipuncture, obtain 3 ml of blood, and carefully dispense the blood into a 13 × 100 mm glass test tube.
2. Place the tube into the 37°C water bath. Allow the blood to clot undisturbed.
3. Allow 30 minutes for the blood to clot and then inspect the clot at 1, 2, 4, and 24 hours, for a retracted clot. Observe the *retraction* of the clot. Record as no retraction, partial retraction, or complete retraction, at each period of inspection. Observe the *appearance* of the clot at the end of the 24 hour period. Record as firm or soft. Also observe for evidence of hemolysis.
4. If a Lee-White clotting time was performed, use tube no. 3 and check for clot retraction at 1, 2, 4, and 24 hours after the blood clotted. Record the results as previously indicated.

Discussion

1. In normal blood, clot retraction should be almost complete within four hours.
2. The clot should be firm. The presence of hemolysins may cause the clot to be soft or partially dissolved.
3. If the blood was carefully drawn, hemolysis should not occur in normal blood samples. Hemolyzed samples should be repeated. If hemolysis occurs during the repeated test, the blood should be examined for hemolysins. The same blood sample may be used to test for clot lysis. If the clot that was initially formed becomes fluid in less than 72 hours, abnormal clot lysis is present.

THE PROTHROMBIN TIME

The prothrombin time is a useful screening procedure to detect deficiencies in the extrinsic system of coagulation; deficiencies of factors II, VII, V, X, and I. Platelet factor 3 is not screened for in the prothrombin time test. When plasma is removed following centrifugation, most of the platelets remain layered on top of the red blood cells. This test is the preferred test used to monitor coumarin drug anitcoagulation therapy. Coumarin drugs inhibit the synthesis of factors II, VII, IX, and X (the prothrombin family). The level of factor VII is the first to decrease following coumarin therapy, with factor II being the last to decrease. Other common causes of a prolonged prothrombin time include vitamin K deficiency and liver disease.

Dr. Armand J. Quick designed the prothrombin time based on his own theory of coagulation in 1935. Since that time he and other researchers have studied the mysteries of coagulation, giving us the theories of today.

The prothrombin time test has been improved since the early days of Dr. Quick, due mainly to the manufacture of reagents that have made the test simple and practical to perform. Several companies produce reagents used in prothrombin time testing. The technologist should *always* follow the manufacturer's instructions that accompany the specific reagents used.

The Principle

Calcium in the blood sample is bound by sodium citrate or sodium oxalate when it is drawn, thus coagulation is prevented. The plasma is removed following centrifugation. Thromboplastin, to which calcium has been added, is mixed with the plasma, and the clotting time is recorded. Normal values range between 10 and 12 seconds. Test conditions vary in different laboratories. Recommended procedure is for each laboratory to establish its own normal range. The technologist should refer to the manufacturer's instructions that accompany the reagents used prior to performing the test.

One-state Prothrombin Time of Quick (Modified)

Equipment and Reagents

1. thromboplastin or thromboplastin reagent (dried)
2. calcium chloride, 0.02M
3. 0.1M sodium oxalate or 3.8% sodium citrate
4. control plasmas (normal and abnormal)
5. 37°C water bath or heat block
6. 13 X 100 mm test tubes
7. stopwatch with second hand
8. pipets

Manual Tilt-Tube Procedure

1. Mix nine parts of freshly collected patient's blood with one part 0.1M sodium oxalate or 3.8% sodium citrate.
2. Centrifuge five minutes at 2000 rpm as soon as possible. Immediately remove plasma to another tube and keep refrigerated until ready to test.
3. 0.02M calcium chloride and thromboplastin are mixed according to the manufacturer's directions. Mix contents thoroughly. If thromboplastin

reagent (dried) is used, reconstitute with the correct amount of distilled water.

4. Pipet 0.2 ml of the thromboplastin-calcium chloride mixture into each of the desired number of 13 × 100 mm test tubes.
5. Warm tubes at 37°C for at least one minute. Warm a small amount of test plasma at 37°C for one minute.
6. Forcibly blow 0.1 ml of test plasma into the prewarmed thromboplastin-calcium chloride mixture and simultaneously start stopwatch.
7. Quickly shake tube (gently) and then hold in water bath without agitation until two or three seconds before clot is expected. It is recommended that all tests be run in triplicate. Timing of first test will be approximate. The second and third tests should check.
8. To read: Wipe tube and hold toward an adequate source of light. Tilt tube very gently once or twice and observe for appearance of a fibrin clot, which is the end point. Stop the watch at this point.

Fibrometer Procedure

1. Mix the thromboplastin and 0.02M calcium chloride according to manufacturer's directions; mix thoroughly. Or, reconstitute thromboplastin reagent (dried) with the correct amount of distilled water.
   With the automatic pipet switched OFF:
2. Place sufficient cups in pre-warmed heat block for the number of tests to be performed. Place tubes of plasmas to be tested into dry wells in rear of heat block. Test plasmas should warm for five minutes, *no longer than ten.*
3. Pipet 0.2 ml of the thromboplastin-calcium chloride mixture into each of the desired number of cups in the heat block.
4. Warm the cups for at least one minute.
   With automatic pipet switched ON:
5. Dispense 0.1 ml of test plasma into cup in reaction well.
6. Machine will start automatically when test plasma is added and stop when fibrin web is formed.
7. Record time, remove and discard cup. Wipe electrodes clean with tissue.

Notes on Procedure

1. Glassware should be scrupulously clean and restricted for prothrombin time determination only.
2. Exact proportions of anticoagulant to blood must be used.
3. Pipets must be wiped clean before returning to their respective tubes. Use of contaminated solutions may result in erroneous prothrombin times.
4. *Rigid standardization of all the details of this test is imperative in order to obtain reproducible and accurate results.*
5. Almost all coagulation procedures have been established using a 37°C waterbath. If dry heat is used, incubation times will have to be reestablished to compensate for its slower conductivity. Even 0.2 ml amounts may take eight minutes to reach 37°C in dry heat as compared to 90 seconds in a waterbath.

Quality Control

1. Normal human plasma (or a commercial plasma) should be used as a control with each series of tests. The control material should be run in the same manner as the test samples. A range of allowable variation should be established for control values within each laboratory. This range usually is based on ±2.0 to ±2.5 standard deviations from the mean control value.
2. It is highly recommended that laboratories establish similar control values for the abnormal range using suitable controls, which may be purchased from a manufacturer of coagulation control reagents.

Limitations of Procedure

Those evaluating prothrombin time testing should be aware of the fact that many commonly administered drugs may affect the results obtained. This should be kept in mind especially when unusual or unexpected abnormal results are obtained. Unexpected abnormal results should always be followed by further coagulation studies to determine the source of the abnormality.

Expected Values

Normal values vary from laboratory to laboratory depending on the technique used.

Discussion

1. Some laboratories report the results of the prothrombin time as the percent of activity. An activity curve is established by making multiple dilutions of the normal plasma control with 0.85% sodium chloride and running a prothrombin time on each dilution. The results are plotted on a graph, the time on the ordinate (vertical) axis and the percent concentration of the control plasma dilution on the abscissa (horizontal) axis. A separate curve must be available for each normal plasma control value. The patient's prothrombin time is then referred to the curve in order to obtain the percent activity of the patients' prothrombin time. The report includes the normal control value in seconds, the patient's prothrombin time in seconds, and the percent activity of the patient's prothrombin time. The actual value of reporting the percent activity is questionable and is not recommended by many of the reagent manufacturers. As a result, many laboratories are not currently using this reporting system. The inconvenience of having to establish curves with each lot of thromboplastin-calcium chloride mixture, the discrepancies from laboratory to laboratory due to different materials and reagents, and the confusion of interpreting the results are among the reasons for eliminating percent activity reporting.
2. A normal and abnormal control must be run with each group of tests performed, and each time a new bottle of thromboplastin is used.
3. It is very important that the thromboplastin-calcium chloride reagent be well mixed before using it in the testing procedure. It is not a homogenous mixture, thus mixing is necessary.

4. The prothrombin time should be performed within 2 hours of collection. *The plasma must be removed from the cellular elements within 30 minutes of collection.* The removed plasma is then kept refrigerated until tested. The plasma may be frozen and stored up to one week without appreciable effect on the prothrombin time.

THE ACTIVATED PARTIAL THROMBOPLASTIN TIME

The activated partial thromboplastin time (APTT) is a useful screening procedure to detect deficiencies in the intrinsic system of coagulation (factors XII, XI, IX, VIII, X, V, II, and I). Platelet factor 3 is not measured since platelet-poor plasma is used.

The Principle

Calcium is removed from the blood sample by the anticoagulant. Following centrifugation, the plasma (minus calcium and platelets) is removed. A platelet substitute (phospholipid), calcium, and an activator are added to the plasma and the time required for coagulation to occur is recorded. Normal values are usually less than 40 seconds. The technologist should refer to the manufacturer's instructions that accompany the reagents used prior to performing the test.

Equipment and Reagents

1. activated partial thromboplastin reagent
2. calcium chloride, 0.02M
3. 3.8% sodium citrate or 0.1M sodium oxalate
4. commercial controls
5. water bath at 37°C or equivalent heat block
6. 13 × 100 mm test tubes
7. stopwatch with second hand
8. pipets

Manual Tilt Tube and Fibrometer Procedure

1. Combine nine parts of freshly collected blood with one part 3.8% sodium citrate or 0.1M sodium oxalate.
2. Mix well. Centrifuge at 3000 rpm for five minutes as soon as possible. Remove supernatant plasma immediately and store in a refrigerator until ready to test. Plasma should be tested within two hours after collection and should not stand at 37°C for more than five minutes.
3. Place tube of 0.02M calcium chloride in 37°C water bath.
4. Pipet 0.1 ml of activated partial thromboplastin into desired number of tubes and place in 37°C water bath. Allow to incubate for a minimum of one minute.
5. Add 0.1 ml plasma (unknown or control) to one activated partial thromboplastin tube. Mix well and allow to incubate at 37°C for two minutes.
   Note: The minimum activation time for the partial thromboplastin-plasma mixture is two minutes. (If using Fibrometer, activation time should be at least three minutes.) Incubation times over five

minutes may cause a loss of Factor V (labile factor) or Factor VIII (AHF) and are not recommended.

6. Forcibly blow 0.1 ml of 0.02M calcium chloride into the activated partial thromboplastin-plasma mixture; simultaneously start stopwatch.

7. Incubate tube in 37°C water bath for 20 seconds. Remove tube and observe for clot formation.
   Note: When times are longer than normal, dip the reaction tube in and out of the water bath to maintain the 37°C temperature while continuing to observe for clot formation.

Quality Control

1. For best results, Fibrometer probes should be washed with a forceful stream of distilled water or saline and wiped dry between determinations to prevent carryover of activated plasma proteins.

2. A control should be run with each series of tests. The control material should be run in the same manner as the test sample. A range of allowable variation should be established for controls in each laboratory. This usually is based on $\pm$ 2.0 to $\pm$ 2.5 standard deviations (S.D.) from the mean control value.

3. Quality control of the activated partial thromboplastin time using control plasmas is used to monitor day-to-day performance of the test system. Interpretation of patient data should always be done in conjunction with the established normal range of the test as outlined in the expected values section of the package insert. Chapter 10 has additional information about maintaining the accuracy of coagulation test results.

Results

1. Results of the activated partial thromboplastin time testing should be reported as the APTT in seconds. These results should be related to the normal range for APTT testing in each laboratory. It is suggested that the patient results be reported to the clinician in conjunction with the normal range. Control values for the reagent test system should never be used in place of a normal range. Furthermore, the reporting of APTT results in terms of an upper normal only may result in incorrect interpretation. Shortened APTT results may also indicate some abnormal condition in the patient's coagulation system.

2. Normal ranges for other populations such as pediatric groups should also be established where warranted. The normal range is usually set $\pm$ 2 or $\pm$ 3 S.D. from the mean value obtained with APTT test on normal individuals under laboratory conditions. Normal ranges may be established on normal healthy individuals as stated under expected values.

Expected Values

1. Since mean values and standard deviations vary from laboratory to laboratory, it is imperative that each laboratory establish a mean value and a normal range for the partial thromboplastin time. The value

and range should be reviewed and revised, when necessary, at regular intervals. In selecting population distributions for establishing the normal range, certain factors should be kept in mind such as age, sex, and the use of individuals that are medication-free versus those who are receiving drugs. In certain instances, a normal population may include individuals who are utilizing commonly accepted drugs such as contraceptive agents. The decision to include such persons in the normal range is at the discretion of the particular laboratory.

2. The following procedure is suggested for establishing the normal range: Using a suitable population of 25-40 normal healthy adults, collect blood into either citrate or oxalate by the same method used for patient samples. The activated partial thromboplastin time should be determined on each normal plasma. The mean and ± 2 standard deviations are calculated.

Discussion

1. An activator (celite, allegic acid, or kaolin) is present in the APTT reagent. This substance is included to insure maximum activation of the contact factors and gives more reproducible results. Without the activator, the clotting time would be greatly increased. The partial thromboplastin time (PTT) is performed exactly the same as the APTT, only without the activator in the reagent. Normal values for the PTT range to 100 seconds.
2. The platelet substitute (a phospholipid) is contained in the APTT reagent or is added to the plasma during the test. The phospholipid is necessary to replace platelet factor 3, which is absent from the plasma of a centrifuged specimen.
3. The APTT and PTT are much more sensitive to coagulation factor deficiencies than is the whole blood clotting time.
4. The APTT does not test for Factor VII or platelet deficiencies. It is sensitive to circulating coagulation inhibitors.
5. The plasma must be removed from the cellular elements within 30 minutes of collection. It is then kept refrigerated until tested and should be tested within two hours for accurate results.

THROMBIN TIME

The thrombin time is a qualitative test for fibrinogen.

The Principle

A thrombin titer is rapidly determined. The fibrin clot formed is proportional to the amount of fibrinogen present. In the absence of fibrinogen, no fibrin clot will form, but if a decreased amount of fibrinogen is present, a small clot that ultimately shrinks will be seen. Normal fibrinogen levels of 150-400 mg/dl will produce a fibrin clot that remains firm for at least 20 minutes. Normal thrombin time is 15-20 seconds. Refer to the manufacturer's instructions accompanying the reagents used prior to performing the test.

Equipment and Reagents

1. thrombin 1,000 units per ml (Parke, Davis & Company): 1 ml of saline is added to a vial containing 1,000 units thrombin per ml
2. tris buffer
3. normal and patient's citrated plasmas
4. pipets
5. 13 × 100 mm test tubes
6. wire loop
7. water bath, 37°C
8. stopwatch

Procedure (Manual Tilt Tube or Wire Loop)

1. 0.2 ml of patient's plasma (or normal plasma) is added to a test tube.
2. Add 0.2 tris buffer to the tube, mix, incubate at 37°C for one minute.
3. Pipet 0.2 ml thrombin solution into the tube, simultaneously starting the stop watch.
4. Dip wire loop through the mixture until a clot is formed. Stop the watch and record the time.
5. Repeat the procedure with the normal control.

Discussion

1. A clotting time of 15 to 20 seconds is normal.
2. The test is sensitive to the presence of fibrinolysins (substances that dissolve fibrin).
3. Low fibrinogen levels may be inherited or acquired. Inherited hypofibrinogenemia is a rare occurrence. Acquired hypofibrinogenemia can be caused by obstetrical accidents such as abruptio placentae or amnionic fluid embolism, causing intravascular clotting, which will result in depletion of fibrinogen.

THROMBOPLASTIN GENERATION TEST

The thromboplastin generation test measures the efficiency with which plasma thromboplastin is formed. The test serves the same basic function as the partial thromboplastin time. If platelets are used as the partial thromboplastin in the incubating mixture, this test can be used to evaluate platelet function.

The Principle

A mixture of deprothrombinized plasma, serum, partial thromboplastin, and calcium are allowed to incubate. When this incubated mixture is added to plasma, rapid clotting occurs. The test consists of an incubation step and a clotting time determination.

*Procedure**

Dilute absorbed plasma (provides the source of factors V, VIII, XI and XII), patient's diluted serum (provides source of factors VII, IX, X, XI and XII), partial thromboplastin (or patient's platelets), and calcium are incubated together. At time intervals up to 6 minutes, a sample of the incubating mixture is added to normal patient plasma and the clotting time is determined.

Discussion

1. The shortest clotting time that is obtained is the thromboplastin generation time.
2. If any of the six tubes has a clotting time of 12 seconds or less within the 6-minute incubation of the generation mixture, the test is considered normal.
3. The presence of circulating anticoagulants will yield abnormal results.

FIBRINOLYTIC ACTIVITY TESTS

Fibrinolysis (the dissolution of fibrin) depends upon the action of the enzyme, plasmin. Plasmin is the proteolytic activated form of plasminogen, one of the plasma proteins. Plasminogen activation is triggered simultaneously with the clotting process. The amount of plasmin formed at any one time is dependent upon the complex and constantly changing balance effected by activator factors and inhibitory factors.

Measurement of the fibrinolytic activity of blood is sometimes useful in detecting abnormalities of this delicate balancing system of activators and inhibitors. Only two tests are discussed in this section of this chapter. The reader is urged to consult a coagulation reference book for additional information and test procedures that deal with this topic.

Euglobulin Lysis Time

The euglobulin fraction of plasma contains fibrinogen and all the plasminogen activators and plasminogen of plasma but only small amounts of the antiplasmins.

The Principle

The lysis of a fibrin clot formed by the addition of thrombin is a measure of the fibrinolytic activity. The euglobulin lysis time is considered a measure of the activator and plasmin activity. Normal clots require more than 2 hours for complete lysis to take place.

Equipment and Reagents

1. citrated blood
2. calcium chloride, 0.025M

---

*Refer to the manufacturer's procedure for the exact steps in performance of the thromboplastin generation test.

3. 1% acetic acid
4. borate solution, pH 9.0
    sodium chloride 9.0g
    sodium borate 1.0g
    dilute to 100 ml distilled water
5. test tubes
6. water bath, 37°C

Procedure

1. Pipet 9.0 ml of distilled water, 0.5 ml patient's plasma, and 0.1 ml 1% acetic acid into a test tube.
2. Refrigerate for 30 minutes at 4°C to allow euglobulin precipitation.
3. Centrifuge at 3,000 RPM for 5 minutes.
4. Decant supernatant and drain tube onto filter paper.
5. Add 0.5 ml of borate solution to precipitate. Place in waterbath and stir gently for 5-10 minutes.
6. Add 0.5 ml of 0.025M calcium chloride to the mixture, start timer, and observe clot formation. Record time.
7. Incubate tube in waterbath; periodically check for clot lysis. When lysis begins, check the tube every 5 minutes until lysis is complete.
8. Report results as the length of time from clot formation to complete lysis of the clot.

Discussion

1. A normal control should always be run for comparison.
2. Pathological fibrinolysis can produce lysis times as short as 5-10 minutes.
3. Platelets prolong the lysis time with their antiplasmin and antiplasminogen activator functions.
4. If the sample is not drained well, antiplasmins will drain back into the precipitate causing prolonged lysis times.

Protamine Sulfate Test

The protamine sulfate test detects the presence of fibrin monomers. When thrombin acts on fibrinogen, fibrin monomers are formed that polymerize to form fibrin. This procedure also detects early fibrin (and fibrinogen) split products. During the process of fibrinolysis, plasmin breaks down fibrin (and fibrinogen) to fragments. During pathological conditions, intravascular coagulation may be stimulated, which results in fibrin deposition in the microcirculation and the appearance of fibrin monomers in the plasma. There is also stimulation of the fibrinolytic process resulting in fibrin (and fibrinogen) split products. Detection of fibrin monomers is therefore important in the diagnosis of disseminated intravascular coagulation (D.I.C.). The procedure for this test is not included in this manual. Refer to the manufacturer's instructions that accompany the reagents used in the protamine sulfate test.

COAGULATION FACTOR DEFICIENCY IDENTIFICATION STUDIES

If abnormal results are obtained from the prothrombin time and activated partial thromboplastin time tests, a coagulation factor deficiency is suspected. However, without additional testing, the exact deficiency (or deficiencies) cannot be determined. Factor identification studies may be useful in identifying bleeding disorders caused by single factor deficiencies.

The Principle

The principle of the studies is to repeat the abnormal test (prothrombin time or APTT) with the addition of two reagents (one reagent to each test repeated). The reagent containing the deficient factor should bring the patient's abnormal time back to a normal time.

Factor Identification Procedure

Equipment and Reagents

1. thromboplastin or thromboplastin reagent (dried)
2. activated partial thromboplastin reagent
3. calcium chloride, 0.02M
4. adsorbed plasma reagent
5. serum reagent
6. 3.8% sodium citrate
7. commercial controls
8. 37°C waterbath or equivalent heat block
9. 13 × 100 mm test tubes
10. stopwatch, with second hand, or suitable instrument
11. pipets

Procedure

1. Mix nine parts of freshly collected patient blood with one part of anticoagulant solution.
2. As soon as possible centrifuge for five minutes at 2,000 rpm. Immediately remove plasma to another tube and keep refrigerated until tested within 2 hours.
3. Reconstitute the thromboplastin reagent (dried) or prepare the thromboplastin-calcium chloride mixture.
4. Reconstitute one vial each of adsorbed plasma reagent, serum reagent, and commercial control.
5. Perform a prothrombin time and an APTT on the patient's plasma and on the control plasma. If the patient's prothrombin time and/or APTT are abnormal, proceed to step 6.
6. "Correct" the patient's plasma as follows:
   a. Add one part patient plasma to one part adsorbed plasma reagent (e.g. 0.5 ml and 0.5 ml).
   b. Add one part patient plasma to one part serum reagent.
7. Using these "corrected" plasmas, repeat the test, or tests found abnormal in step 5.

TABLE II
CORRECTION STUDIES

Patient's Original Time		APTT		Prothrombin Time		
APTT	PT	Plasma Reagent	Serum Reagent	Plasma Reagent	Serum Reagent	Deficiency Indicated
N	N	-	-	-	-	No deficiency
A	N	C	NC	-	-	VIII
A	N	C	C	-	-	XI, XII*
A	N	NC	C	-	-	IX
A	A	C	NC	C	NC	V
A	A	NC	C	NC	C	X
A	A	NC	NC	NC	NC	II
N	A	-	-	NC	C	VII

Key:
N = Normal time
A = Abnormal time
C = Time corrected to normal
- = Not applicable
NC = Time not corrected to normal

Interpretation

1. The prolonged glass clotting time of XII deficiency distinguishes it from the relatively normal glass clotting time of an XI deficiency.
2. For the patient's abnormal APTT to be considered corrected, the time on the patient's "corrected" plasma must be within the normal range for the technique and reagents used.
3. For the patient's abnormal prothrombin time to be considered corrected, the time on the "corrected" plasma must be 15 seconds or less.

Discussion

1. If the patient's APTT is normal and the prothrombin time is abnormal, it can be assumed that a factor VII deficiency is present and no identification studies are necessary.
2. The adsorbed plasma reagent contains coagulation factors I, V, VIII, XI, and XII. Other factors have been adsorbed by barium sulfate.
3. The serum reagent contains coagulation factors VII, IX, X, XI, and XII. Other coagulation factors were consumed during coagulation. A serum reagent may be easily prepared in the laboratory. However, it is important to obtain serum from 6-8 persons in order to be assured of having a serum reagent with high levels of the proper coagulation factors.

FACTOR ASSAY

Factor assays are performed to determine the concentration of the particular factor that is found to be deficient. The amount and type of therapy given will depend upon which factor is deficient and the degree (or amount) of the deficiency. Assays of the factors are performed using the test system that detects abnormalities in the specific coagulation pathway where the factor is involved, i.e. intrinsic or extrinsic.

A normal curve is established by making serial dilutions of normal plasma from 1:5 to 1:320 in a buffer. A factor deficient plasma (the deficient plasma contains high levels of all factors except the specific one for which the curve is being established) is added 1:1 to each of the serial dilutions and the appropriate test (APTT or prothrombin time) is run on each dilution. The times are plotted on two-cycle log-log graph paper with the percent dilution on the abscissa and seconds on the ordinate. A 1:5 dilution of the patient's abnormal plasma is prepared with the buffer and is added 1:1 to the factor deficient plasma. The appropriate test (APTT or prothrombin time) is run on the patient's plasma-factor deficient plasma mixture. The percent of deficiency is found by locating the point on the ordinate where the patient's time intercepts the normal curve and reading the percent deficiency from the abscissa. The reader is referred to the insert sheet accompanying the reagents for additional information and exact instructions for performing a factor assay.

PLATELET FUNCTION TESTS

In Vivo Platelet Adhesion

In vivo adhesion to collagen is an important part of the platelets' function in hemostasis. It has been extremely difficult to assess this function in vitro. Several in vitro tests have been devised in which platelet retention to glass beads in a column has been measured. Due to the variability in components, these techniques are difficult to standardize. The nonphysiological environment of the glass bead column is also a subject of controversy in the assessment of the in vivo platelet function. The method of Borchgrevink has some merit in the measurement of platelet in vivo ability to adhere to a surface. This manual will include only this procedure for the measurement of platelet adhesiveness.

Borchgrevink Method

Principle

When a vessel is damaged or cut, there is almost immediate adhesion of the platelets to the site of the injury. The Borchgrevink method is based on determining the difference between the platelet count in a venous blood sample and the platelet count from the last of the series of counts from a capillary incision. Theoretically, some platelets will adhere to the collagen surrounding the incision and fewer and fewer platelets will be found in the drops of blood as time progresses. Normal values: 24%-58% adhesive platelets.

Equipment and Reagents

1. phase counting chamber, No. 1 coverslips
2. phase microscope
3. erythrocyte diluting pipets and aspirator
4. siliconized test tubes

5. 1% ammonium oxalate in distilled water, filtered
6. siliconized or plastic syringe for venipuncture
7. the template system as for the bleeding time
8. petri dishes, wet cotton gauze pads

Procedure

1. Make a standard incision of the skin as for the bleeding time determination.
2. Allow the blood to flow undisturbed until the drop is large enough to fill the red cell diluting pipet for a phase platelet count (or regular platelet count if phase microscopy is unavailable).
3. After 1 minute fill another pipet and each minute thereafter until bleeding ceases. *Do not disturb the incision.* Excess blood may be removed by blotting with filter paper.
4. A platelet count is performed on the last capillary pipet sample.
5. By venipuncture, withdraw a blood sample using a siliconized syringe and place the blood in a siliconized test tube with EDTA anticoagulant. A dilution of the venous blood is made using the red cell pipet.
6. A platelet count is performed on the venous sample.
7. Calculate the percent adhesiveness as follows:

$$\% \ adhesiveness = \frac{\begin{array}{c} platelet \ count \\ in \ venous \ blood \end{array} - \begin{array}{c} platelet \ count \\ in \ last \ capillary \ pipet \end{array}}{platelet \ count \ in \ venous \ blood} \times 100$$

Discussion

1. Decreased platelet adhesiveness is seen in von Willebrand's disease, thrombasthenia, macroglobulinemia, azotemia, myelofibrosis, Storage Pool deficiencies, multiple myeloma, and drug-induced platelet dysfunction syndromes.
2. Standardization of technique is difficult to control unless utmost care is taken to maintain uniformity in the procedures. Meaningful results, when combined with the bleeding time, may serve as the best tool to substantiate a diagnosis of von Willebrand's disease.
3. Each laboratory should determine its own set of normal values as with most other procedures.

Platelet Aggregation

Platelet aggregation is defined as the adherence of one platelet to another. The ability of platelets to adhere to each other is ultimately important in the formation of the platelet thrombus or plug prior to fibrin formation. Born and Cross observed that the optical density of platelet-rich plasma, less that of platelet-free plasma, was proportional to the concentration of platelets. This observation was the basis for their turbidimetric method for continuously recording platelet aggregation in platelet-rich plasma. When aggregation occurs, platelets clump together and thus the number of platelets occurring as separate particles decreases and the light transmission increases. This change is measured spectrophotometrically and a tracing is made with a recorder.

Principle

An aggregating agent (ADP, collagen, epinephrine, ristocetin, thrombin) is added to the platelet-rich plasma that is constantly being stirred. As the platelets aggregate, the plasma becomes progressively clearer. An optical system detects the change in light transmission, and a recorder graphically records the variations in light transmissions from a baseline setting.

Equipment and Reagents

1. aggregometer and recorder
2. appropriate cuvettes with Teflon®-coated magnetic stir bars
3. plastic test tubes
4. pipets:
   a. plastic, 1 ml serological
   b. 20 μl, with disposable tips
5. 3.8% sodium citrate solution
6. 0.85% sodium chloride solution
7. veronal buffer, pH 7.3.
8. ADP:
   a. stock solution: 507 mg ADP in 50 ml veronal buffer. Freeze 1 ml aliquots.
   b. working solutions: Prepare just prior to use. Dilute 1:5 and 1:10 with veronal buffer.
9. epinephrine: Adrenaline hydrochloride (1 mg/ml).
   a. Dilute 1:10 with veronal buffer.
10. collagen: Soluble skin collagen. Each bottle label gives mg/ml of collagen. Dilute with saline to obtain a concentration of approximately 0.08 mg/ml of collagen.
11. thrombin (human):
    a. stock solution: Reconstitute 50 units of thrombin with 1 ml saline.
    b. working solution: Dilute 0.1 ml stock with 0.56 ml saline.
12. ristocetin: Dissolve 100 mg in 4 ml saline. Store frozen. Thaw just before use.

Procedure

1. Withdraw 9 ml blood in a plastic syringe into 1 ml sodium citrate. Centrifuge 30 minutes at 150 G at *room temperature* to prepare platelet-rich plasma (PRP). Carefully aspirate plasma with a plastic pipet. Store in a covered plastic tube at *room temperature*. The tests should be performed within 2 hours. Platelet-poor plasma (PPP) is prepared by further centrifugation at 3,000 G for 20 minutes. Dilute PRP and PPP with equal parts of saline for standardizing the aggregometer setting. Unless the test plasma is lipemic, a water blank may be used in place of the PPP. Normal plasma should be run along with the patient.

2. Add diluted PRP to cuvette and adjust the *Bias* as indicated in the instructions that accompany the aggregometer. Place PPP in a cuvette and insert in the aggregometer; adjust the Gain according to instrument instructions. Perform the tests with the various aggregating agents. Reset the aggregometer if necessary before each test.

3. Aggregation tests:
   a. Dilute 0.25 ml PRP with 0.25 saline in cuvette. Add stir bar and place in aggregometer for 2 minutes to reach 37°C. Record a baseline for approximately 1 minute.
   b. Add 20 μl of aggregating agent. Dispense into middle of tube.
   c. Record results for approximately 3-5 minutes, or until no further changes occur.
   d. Repeat with each of 5 aggregating agents.

Discussion

1. Preparation of the platelet-rich plasma is critical. It must be prepared and assayed as soon as possible (no longer than 2 hours after the sample is obtained). The patient or control must abstain from ingestion of aspirin, aspirin-related drugs, and antihistamines for 7 days prior to the test.

2. Plastic equipment must be used for withdrawing, transferring, and storing the blood, plasma, PRP, and PPP.

3. Citrate concentration, pH, and temperature are very important in aggregation and must be carefully controlled.

4. All plasmas should remain at room temperature for approximately 30 minutes before testing. Platelets *should never be heated or refrigerated.*

5. ADP and epinephrine usually produce biphasic curves. The secondary aggregation phase occurs following platelet release of intracellular ADP and epinephrine. This is critical to measuring platelet secretion (Figure 40). Aspirin, and aspirin-containing compounds, antihistamines, etc., cause reduced aggregation, especially in the secondary phase.

6. Collagen produces a lag phase, then a monophasic curve. Thrombin has a monophasic curve and frequently produces clot formation in

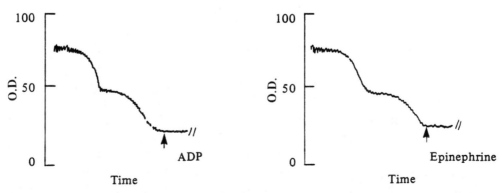

Figure 40. Aggregation of normal platelets by ADP and epinephrine (optimum concentration).

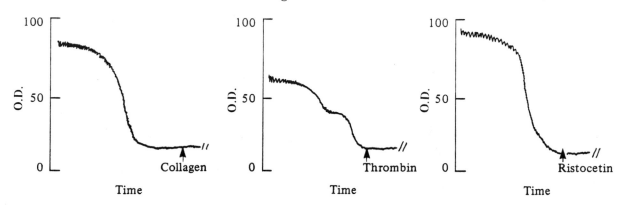

Figure 41. Aggregation of platelets by collagen, thrombin, and ristocetin.

strong dilutions, and disaggregation in weak dilutions. Ristocetin produces biphasic curves which are usually obscured and appear monophasic. (Figure 41). Von Willebrand's disease produces no aggregation with ristocetin, while other agents remain normal. Ristocetin-induced aggregation may be restored to normal upon the addition of normal plasma in von Willebrand's disease.

7. Serotonin may also be used as an aggregating agent. Aggregation proceeds to 10%-30% transmittance, then disaggregation occurs.
8. In Glanzmann's disease, aggregation is induced *only with ristocetin.*
9. Many variables affect platelet aggregation in addition to disease and drugs mentioned previously. The amount of exercise, emotional stress, smoking, and dietary fat intake prior to the test may produce variable degrees of hyperaggregation. Alcohol tends to stabilize the platelet membrane, thus reducing aggregation.
10. The number of platelets in the PRP is of utmost importance. 50,000/μl are necessary for aggregation with ADP and collagen; 75,000/μl for aggregation with epinephrine.

STUDY QUESTIONS

1. Define:
   a. bleeding time.
   b. coagulation time.
2. What is the value of performing the bleeding time?
3. Give the normal values for the following:
   a. Duke bleeding time _____.
   b. Ivy bleeding time _____.
   c. Capillary coagulation time _____.
   d. Lee-White clotting time _____.
   e. Clot retraction _____.
   f. Prothrombin time _____.
   g. Activated partial thromboplastin time _____.
4. Why is the coagulation time longer than the bleeding time?
5. A prolonged bleeding time would indicate the need for what additional tests?
6. Why does the Mielke template method give a more accurate bleeding time than the Ivy method?

7. Give two reasons why the Lee-White clotting time is longer than the capillary coagulation time.
8. Why is the Lee-White clotting time no longer the method of choice to monitor heparin anticoagulant therapy?
9. What is the value of performing the coagulation time?
10. What are some aspects of qualtity control that must be strictly observed in coagulation studies?
11. In the Ivy bleeding time, the pressure cuff is inflated to _____ mm of mercury.
12. List the reagents used to perform the prothrombin time.
13. Why are the normal values for the prothrombin time and the activated partial thromboplastin time not included with the reagent instructions?
14. What clotting substances are added during the prothrombin time test that are absent from the test plasma?
15. List the reagents used to perform the activated partial thromboplastin time.
16. What clotting substances are added during the activated partial thromboplastin time that are absent from the test plasma?
17. List the two reagents used for factor identification studies and indicate the coagulation factors present in each reagent.
18. Describe the procedure for performing factor identification studies.
19. Identify the deficient factor if the abnormal prothrombin time and the abnormal activated partial thromboplastin time are both corrected by the serum reagent.
20. Identify the deficient factor if the abnormal activated partial thromboplastin time is corrected by the plasma reagent. (PT was normal.)
21. Give a brief description of the procedure for performing factor assays.
22. List the purposes of performing the following tests:
    a. Thrombin Time.
    b. Thromboplastin Generation Test.
    c. Euglobulin Lysis Time.
    d. Protamine Sulfate Test.
23. Define platelet adhesion.
24. What is the principle involved in the Borchgrevink method of measuring in vivo platelet adhesion?
25. Why are glass bead platelet adhesion tests a subject of controversy?
26. List 5 substances used to induce platelet aggregation.
27. List 10 variables that will affect platelet aggregation.
28. Describe the aggregometer tracing induced by the following aggregating agents:
    a. ADP
    b. epinephrine
    c. collagen
    d. ristocetin
    e. thrombin
    f. serotonin

Chapter 10

QUALITY ASSURANCE IN THE CLINICAL LABORATORY

OBJECTIVES

The student will learn and/or identify the following:

1. the meaning of quality assurance.
2. the purpose of quality assurance programs.
3. the goals of quality assurance programs.
4. how to choose a reagent control for a quality assurance program.
5. how to use a control to establish a quality assurance program.
6. how to calculate the mean value and the standard deviation of a control.
7. how to identify shifts in the confidence limits.
8. how to identify trends in the confidence limits.
9. how to utilize a Levey-Jennings chart to its fullest potential.
10. how to calculate the coefficient of variation.
11. additional measures of quality assurance.

INTRODUCTION

From the beginning it became evident to those involved in the clinical laboratory that in order to increase confidence in laboratory results, some evidence of its reliability had to be available. This evidence would help the physician have more confidence in the data he received and, as he realized the benefit of these results, his usage of laboratory tests would increase; the laboratory would grow and become an intricate part of the health facilities. This indeed has been the case. The evidence of reliability referred to has become the Quality Assurance Programs we know today.

QUALITY ASSURANCE

Quality Assurance has become such a part of the clinical laboratory that pathologists and technologists generally will not consider new laboratory procedures unless some means of control is available. Large institutions have separate Q.A. departments with at least one technologist whose sole responsibility it is to prepare the Quality Assurance data and budgeting for the entire laboratory. Without an on-going Q.A. program, laboratories would not be allowed to operate today. Quality Assurance is required as a means of evaluation by those regulatory agencies that inspect clinical laboratories.

A Quality Assurance program forms a large part of a laboratory's budget, thus it is not an inexpensive process. It must be used to its full potential. With proper monitoring and interpretation of Q.A. results, a laboratory can not only recognize an out of control situation but also predict it will happen. By using the tools available to them, technologists can take advantage of Q.A. results to identify causes of out of control situations. If "down time" is avoided and/or the length of down time shortened, the laboratory is gaining some monetary value from its Quality Assurance program other than simply meeting regulatory requirements.

The Goals of Quality Assurance Programs

One goal of the laboratory should be to improve its accuracy and precision. It is possible to have precision without accuracy; it is also possible to have accuracy without precision. If the target value of a control is 100 units and on duplicate runs values of 90 and 110 are achieved, there is no precision even though the resulting average is 100. If on the same control values of 89 and 91 are recovered, there is precision, but the average is not accurate. Finally, if the duplicate results are 99 and 101, there is both accuracy and precision.

Choosing a Control for Quality Assurance

It is the responsibility of the laboratory to choose a control for its program that best fits its needs. A control should be capable of responding to variations within the test system similar to the way a patient sample would respond under the same conditions. It is also desirable to have a control that is stable for several weeks or, better yet, for a year. This will allow the day-to-day variability that one might see in a Quality Assurance program to be accurately attributed to variables within the system rather than to variables from lot to lot. The response of a control to system variations that are necessary and the long-life stability that is desirable are not always compatible. Alterations of a control material in an attempt to stabilize it can reduce its ability to respond to system changes.

The art of lypholyzation allows coagulation controls to achieve long-term dating of up to two years. It must be understood that due to lypholyzation the control is not entirely like fresh plasma and should never be substituted for freshly drawn samples. It will, however, respond to changing test conditions that affect accuracy and precision.

Hematology controls are even more difficult to prepare since the cell portions cannot be significantly altered to extend the life beyond 60 days and still achieve good response to variables. Because of this, laboratories have to utilize several lots over the period of one year. This is less desirable but it can be managed.

Using the Control to Establish Quality Assurance

When a laboratory begins a new lot of control in a coagulation program, that control should be tested at least 20 and preferably 30 days. It should be treated as an unknown in the testing system and it should be subjected to all the variables that will exist over that period. These variations would include day-to-day changes in instrumentation, changes in techniques, reconstitution variations, and even "bad Monday-good Friday" attitudes that affect laboratory results. If these conditions are ignored, as would be the case if 30 results were run on one day by one technologist, the allowable range would be too narrow. In this case, the laboratory would have more bad control results than good in the future utilization of the program.

Calculating the Mean and Standard Deviation

After the 30 control results are available the mean and standard deviation are calculated. The mean is the average of the 30 results.
The formula is:

$$\bar{X} = \Sigma \div N$$

where Σ = sum of values
N = number of values
$\bar{X}$ = mean

Next the Standard Deviation (S.D.) is calculated as a way of measuring the dispersion of a group of data, in this case the 30 values. S.D. equals the square root of the sum of the squared differences between the mean and each individual value divided by the number of values minus one.
The formula is:

$$S.D. = \frac{\sqrt{\Sigma (X_1 - \bar{X})^2}}{n-1}$$

The laboratory usually applies the mean and S.D. to what is called a Levey-Jennings chart. One can look at this chart as a Gaussian Curve lying on its side. See example and Figure 42.

Example: Prothrombin Time Control Mean = 12.0 seconds
1 S.D. = 0.5 seconds

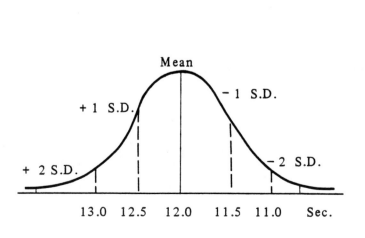
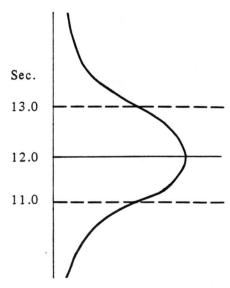

Figure 42. Gaussian curve.

As you will note in Figure 42, a range of ±2 S.D. has been set. Statistically it is calculated that approximately 68% of all values will fall within ±1 S.D., 95.5% within ±2 S.D., and 99% within ±3 S.D. It is generally considered too strict to work within ±1 S.D. and too lenient to work at ±3 S.D. Two S.D. is considered proper and, therefore, one can expect 45 out of every 1000 results to fall outside of ±2 S.D. without any apparent reason. When this happens the control must be repeated. The repeated control should return to within the ±2 S.D. range. The odds are very high against the control repeating an out of range value unless something is truly wrong in the test system.

The Levey-Jennings chart is now established as a means of tracking the progress of this particular test. Each day a control is run and the result is plotted on the chart. The plotted points are connected with a line and shortly a chart such as Figure 43 develops.

Shifts in the Confidence Limits

The 2 S.D. lines are sometimes called confidence limits. To accept everything within these lines as status quo is not using the Levey-Jennings chart to its fullest potential. One should expect to see over a period of days an equal scattering of results above and below the mean as seen in Figure 43. If this does not occur, then it should be a warning that something is not proper in the system. Statistically, no more than 6 values should fall on one side of the mean in succession. If this occurs, it is considered *a shift*. (See Figure 44). It can usually be attributed to something happening on one day that has moved all values high or low. The results may still be within the confidence limits but the test is out of control and should be investigated as soon as possible. Possible causes of a shift could be the changing of a lamp

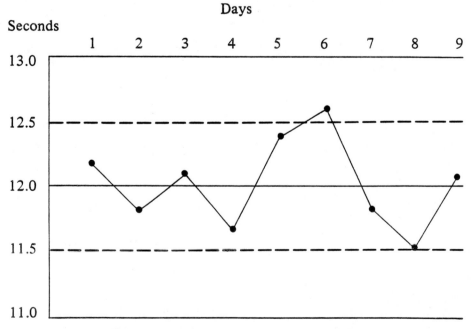

Figure 43. Levey-Jennings chart, plotted, 9 days.

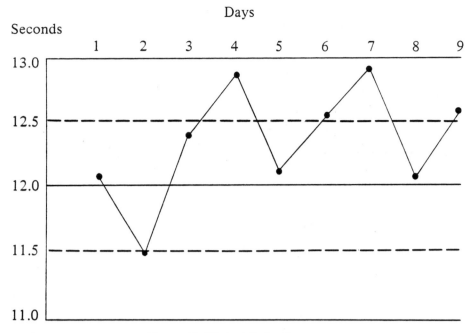

Figure 44. High shift in the mean.

in the instrument, damaging the instrument probe, or changing the lot of reagent.

Trends in the Confidence Limits

Out of control situations may not happen suddenly but may occur gradually over a period of days. This is considered *a trend* and should lead one to expect a different set of possible causes. (See Figure 45.) Again the results are within the confidence limits but it is a warning of things to come if some attention is not directed to the system. Possible causes could be a deteriorating reagent, a changing heat supply, deteriorating lamp, or anything that would lend itself to gradual change.

Using the Levey-Jennings Chart to Its Fullest Potential

The Levey-Jennings chart should be used like a diary of the particular test for which it is constructed and all alterations in the test system should be noted on it. Such things as reagent lot number changes, instrument service, or adjustment changes are examples. If shifts or trends develop due to these alterations, they can be visually related to the most likely cause. Additionally, if out of control situations are corrected, a note on the chart may aid someone the next time a similar situation occurs. (See Figure 46.)

Quality Assurance in Hematology

Hematology control is generally handled in a similar manner as previously described. The fact that the control has a much shorter shelf-life does not allow the laboratory to work with a mean over a long period of time.

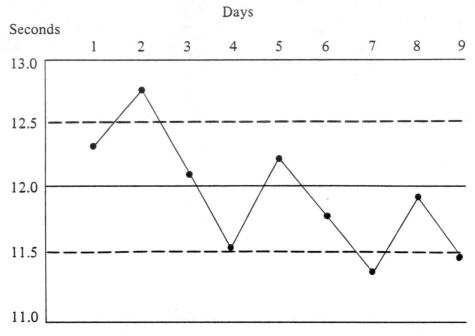

Figure 45. Downward trend.

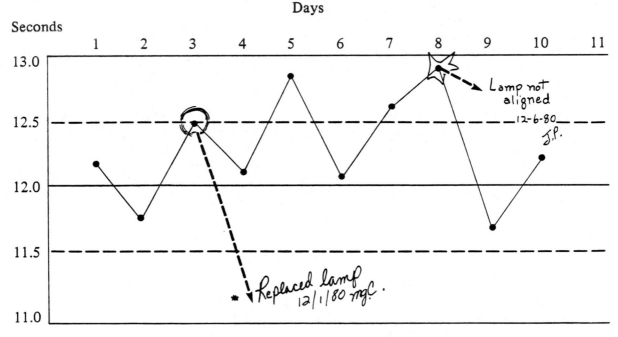

Figure 46. Levey-Jennings chart with changes noted.

Since establishing a mean of 30 values may use up half the shelf-life of the control, generally a target value of 10 results over a period of 2-3 days is used. The S.D. range established on the previous lot of control is applied to this target value if the assay values of the two lots involved are similar, which is usually the case.

Coefficient of Variation

Another calculation that is used in Q.A. programs is the Coefficient of Variation (C.V.). This is especially helpful when short dated controls like hematology are used or where the precision of methods with different means or Standard Deviations is a concern. The C.V. is the percentage expression of the S.D. and is calculated as follows:

$$C.V.(\%) = \frac{S.D.}{\bar{X}} \times 100$$

If laboratory A has a mean of 100 and an S.D. of ±2 and laboratory B has a mean of 200 and an S.D. of ±2, one cannot say that both laboratories have the same precision. Laboratory B has better precision because its C.V. is 1% while laboratory A has a C.V. of 2%. Some laboratories replace S.D. with C.V. when working with short-dated, often changing lot numbers.

Additional Quality Assurance Measures

There are many additional tools that can be used to monitor, record, and evaluate the testing efficiency of a laboratory. These include Histograms, Cumulative Sum Charts, Youden Plots, and t-Test, to name a few. They all have particular values. The limitation of this chapter does not allow for the coverage of all of them. All are worth consideration for certain laboratory needs.

A laboratory must never become so involved with graphs and charts that it loses sight of its ultimate goal: providing the best possible test results. Quality Assurance is more than controls, charts, and records. We can have the best control, accuracy, and precision, the most elaborate charts and graphs, but if the test results are wrong, we have not provided an adequate, reliable service to the patient. Quality Assurance involves proper patient and sample identification, properly handled patient samples, properly maintained equipment, a properly arranged and organized laboratory, and (most importantly) properly educated and dedicated laboratorians.

STUDY QUESTIONS

1. Define Quality Assurance.
2. What are two important goals of any Quality Assurance program?
3. What are two important qualities a laboratory should look for when choosing a control for its Q.A. program?
4. Write the formulas for calculating the following:
   a. the mean
   b. the standard deviation
   c. the coefficient of variation
5. What is the purpose of a Levey-Jennings chart?
6. Define:
   a. shift of the mean
   b. trends in the confidence limits
7. Why should any alterations within a particular test system be noted on the Levey-Jennings chart?
8. List additional measures of Quality Assurance in the laboratory.

REFERENCES

Brown, Barbara: *Hematology: Principles and Procedures*, ed. 2. Lea and Febiger, Philadelphia. 1976.

Davidsohn, Israel and Henry, John: *Todd and Sanford Clinical Diagnosis and Management by Laboratory Methods*, ed. 16, Vol. I. W.B. Saunders, Philadelphia. 1979.

Erslev, Allan and Gabuzda, Thomas G.: *Pathophysiology of Blood*, ed. 2. W.B. Saunders, Philadelphia. 1979.

Fareed, Jawed, Messmore, Harry, and Bermer, Edward W.: New perspectives in coagulation testing. *Clinical Chemistry, 26*: 10, 1980.

Hemostasis Symposium, Dade Division American Hospital Supply Corporation. W. Dundee, Illinois. 1977.

Hutchison, Doug: *Platelet Function, Disorders and Testing*: Dade Monograph. Dade Division American Hospital Supply Corporation, Miami. 1979.

Hyun, Bong, Ashton, John, and Dolan, Kathleen: *Practical Hematology*. W.B. Saunders, Philadelphia. 1975.

Instruction and Service Manual for the Coulter Counter® Model Fn, Coulter Electronics, Florida. 1970.

Lee, Leslie: *Elementary Principles of Laboratory Instruments*, ed. 4. C.V. Mosby, St. Louis. 1978.

Miale, John B.: *Laboratory Medicine: Hematology*, ed. 5. C.V. Mosby, St. Louis. 1977.

Rosalki, S.B. (Ed.): *New Pathways in Laboratory Medicine: Transactions of the Merz + Dade Exploratory Seminar*. Düdingen, Switzerland. Hans Huber, Bern, Switzerland. 1978.

Simmons, Arthur: *Technical Hematology*, ed. 2. J.B. Lippincott, Philadelphia. 1976.

Sirridge, Marjorie: *Laboratory Evaluation of Hemostasis*. Lea & Febiger, Philadelphia. 1974.

Tietz, Norbert W.: *Fundamentals of Clinical Chemistry*, ed. 2. W.B. Saunders, Philadelphia. 1976.

Vollmer, Kay: *Coagulation Procedures*: Dade Monograph. Dade Division American Hospital Supply Corporation, Miami. 1976.

INDEX